Victory Over
ADHD

How a mother's journey to natural medicine
reversed her children's severe emotional,
mental, and behavioral problems.

Deborah Merlin
Larry Cook

EcoVision Communications

Los Angeles, California

Publisher
EcoVision Communications
www.TheNaturalGuide.com

Writers
Deborah Merlin
Larry Cook

Editors
Bobbie Christmas
Kay Neth

Foreword
David R. Allen, MD

Peer Reviewers
Judith Bluestone, Director, The HANDLE Institute
Mary Robson, Clinician, The HANDLE Institute
Billie J. Sahley, PhD

Cover Design
Sandra Busta

Library of Congress Control Number
2005939148

ISBN 0-9755361-7-6 & 978-0-9755361-7-9

Disclaimer

The information presented in this book is not intended to diagnose, treat, cure, or prevent any disease. The information contained herein is designed to educate the reader and is not intended to provide individual medical advice. If you have a medical condition, please consult a licensed health care practitioner.

Dedication

During the most critical phases of my children's health crisis, many professionals offered invaluable advice and support. It's difficult to imagine what might have happened without their wisdom, patience, and guidance. These phenomenal professionals include the NICU staff at Santa Monica Medical Center, social workers, Westside Regional Center, nurses, teachers, special education support teams with the Los Angeles Unified School District, Village Glen West, psychologists, occupational therapists, speech therapists, homeopaths, and medical doctors who practice alternative medicine. Thanks to all of you for helping children (and adults) with special needs.

Acknowledgments

Special Gratitude To:
- My children Erik and Westley for teaching me motherhood on the deepest level.
- My husband, Chris, for having the wisdom to say, "No" to Ritalin and for supporting my mission to write this book.
- My mother, Joan McCausland; father Gordon Reinauer; sister Kathryn Payette; brother-in-law Mark Merlin, PhD; and sister-in-law Sally Merlin Smyth for editing parts of the manuscript and their enthusiasm.
- David R. Allen, MD, for thinking outside the box and healing my children by addressing the cause and not just the symptoms. Additional thanks is due to Dr. Allen for writing the foreword to this book.
- Billie Jay Sahley, PhD, for reading the first draft, valuable suggestions, contributions on amino acids, and a peer review.
- Judith Bluestone and Mary Robson of The HANDLE Institute for their contributions in Chapters 5, 6 and 7 and their peer reviews.
- Jeanne M. Zeeb-Schecter, DHM, and Jack Johnson, PhD, of Q-Metrx, for their contributions to the book.
- My friends Glenna Citron, Sigrid Macdonald, and Katherine Redwine for reading parts of the entire manuscript or all of it, for their suggestions, and for their unconditional love and support.
- All my enlightened woman friends in the wisdom circle.
- Pamela Healey, CN, MHom: thank you for being an advocate for my book and believing so much in it. A very special thank you for connecting me to my publisher.
- Larry Cook, my publisher and editor, for bringing my book to the highest level and for feeling passionate about ADHD/ADD.
- Kay Neth for her invaluable editing.
- Sandra Busta for my beautiful cover.

Please Share With Me

Please let me know how my book has helped you or changed your life; or let me know if you have any questions or feedback. My email is: Deborah@VictoryOverADHD.com.

Contents

Contents

Part 2: ADHD: A Holistic Approach
By Larry Cook & Deborah Merlin

Contents

Contents

Foreword
David R. Allen, MD

An epidemic of problems affects our children in this twenty-first century. We have the usual problems of drug abuse, delinquency, and the uncertainty of the future, but in addition to these important issues, we are faced with an unprecedented rise in autism and ADHD. These complex conditions often overwhelm the average person's ability to understand and therefore seek effective treatment.

As a physician, I have various treatment options for ADHD, autism, and other psychiatric problems in children. The conventional medical treatments consist mainly of various prescription medications. Although effective in some cases, there are many negative side effects that limit their use. However, there are many alternative treatments that don't use drugs or have significant side effects. These alternative approaches may include nutrition improvement; vitamin supplementation; elimination of food known to cause allergies; heavy metal detoxification; the balancing of neurotransmitters by amino acids; acupuncture; and herbs to help address root causes and then strengthen, build, and repair weakened bodily systems. The elimination of candida and parasites from the bowel is often included in alternative treatments, yet ignored by conventional medicine.

I am often shocked by how quickly a child is placed on a medication—such as Ritalin—without the investigation of safe, natural medicine approaches. The need for the education of parents and their children about alternative medicine and lifestyle choices is the reason why I'm enthusiastically writing this foreword for Deborah's story.

Deborah Merlin—mother of two premature infants—had the courage and the tenacity to do everything possible to ensure that her children grew up to be normal, healthy adults. As you will discover, the task was not easy. Westley and Erik, whom I have seen in the clinic, are now wonderful young adults. Their story is an immensely interesting journey through many doctors and philosophies. Deborah has been given conflicting diagnoses, often with opposing suggested treatments, yet she remained steadfast in seeking what made sense to her as a mother. Often the "nonprofessional mother" is more correct than the experts.

This book fills an important need—it's an idea whose time has come. For all the mothers and fathers who are confused and searching, this book will bring clarity. I know this book will open a whole new possibility for the many parents and children who read it.

Chapter 1
From Sickness to Health:
My Children's Journey

If you've picked up this book, you're probably curious about natural living. You want to make healthy choices for you and your family. Maybe you'd like to know more about alternative medicine. Perhaps you have a child with an attention disorder, behavioral difficulties, or neurological problems—and you want solutions.

You've come to the right place.

I spent a great deal of time, energy, and money looking for solutions for my children—two young boys who were diagnosed with attention disorders by the time they were three years old. It would take me *seven years* of searching to find what my children really needed to address their problems. And the solutions had nothing to do with Ritalin or other conventional medical approaches. The answers lay in improving my children's diet, discovering and addressing nutritional deficiencies, and turning to other natural approaches. Along the way, I discovered the health choices that *I* had to make for us to live optimally, healthfully, and happily.

Once I figured out what my boys needed to thrive, the results were dramatic. Exploring natural remedies was well worth my time. But you can begin the healing process faster than I did by using the information and resources in the second part of this book—in addition to my story, a seven-year journey toward health and well-being.

Love, Marriage, and Pregnancy

I was thirty-three years old and single, working as an insurance inspector and living in an apartment in Santa Monica, California. I drove a red MR2 Toyota sports car and worked out at the gym every day. I was having a good time, though my life lacked substance.

I met Chris at the gym one Sunday morning in an aerobics class. We were married thirty-two days after our first date. We were madly in love, and I wanted to get pregnant right away. He wanted to wait two years, so we compromised and decided to start trying to get pregnant in a year. Chris understandably wanted to spend some time alone with me, but I was concerned about my biological clock.

At an ob-gyn appointment, I told my doctor that I planned to start trying to conceive in three months, which would have been June 1. It would take a while, my doctor warned, because I was thirty-four years old.

I conceived on June 4. Unfortunately, conceiving was the only easy thing about my pregnancy.

When I was about six weeks pregnant, I did a light workout at the gym. I went home, took a shower and started to make breakfast. Suddenly, I felt my legs become damp. I looked under my bathrobe—blood was streaming down my legs. In a panic I called my doctor. He told me there was a fifty percent chance that I would miscarry—but the fact that I wasn't experiencing cramps was a good sign.

The next morning, Chris and I went to see the doctor, who, to our relief, determined that I was still pregnant. We scheduled an ultrasound for the following Friday.

That night I dreamed I was back where I grew up on the East Coast, wearing a blue maternity dress, telling my family that I was expecting twins. The following morning I told my husband about the dream. He quickly interrupted me. Twins, Chris groaned, would be his worst nightmare—the extra responsibility, the expense.

The following Friday I went to have the ultrasound while Chris was at work.

The monitor showed two hearts beating.

Twins.

After the ultrasound, my doctor warned me that I would probably have another bleeding episode at three months. A twin pregnancy would be a totally different ballgame, he noted. I would have to stop working at six months and spend the duration of the pregnancy in bed.

I felt a little scared—and excited. But how would Chris react to the news?

When he arrived home, I took him into the bedroom and sat him down. Chris asked me how the ultrasound went. I told him I was still pregnant. And we were going to have twins.

Chris was speechless. He got his voice back twenty-four hours later. Before long he was bragging to everyone that we were expecting two babies, not just one.

As my doctor had predicted, I had a bleeding episode at three months. He also told me that twins tend to be born early, and if I went into premature labor, medicines could stop the contractions, provided I received immediate medical attention.

The second bleeding stopped, and I was doing well. My doctor had nixed exercise. But I continued to work full time, even as I was becoming larger than I ever would've imagined. I looked ridiculous driving a little red sports car.

My last day of work was the day before Thanksgiving. The next day, I didn't feel well. Nonetheless, we drove to my mother-in-law's house for dinner in our brand new station wagon. I ate modestly—but shortly after dinner I felt nauseated. My mother-in-law told me I looked gray. I wanted to go home—to throw up in private. I was sure we could make it to our house in time; we lived just a mile away. But the ride felt like an eternity.

As we pulled into the driveway, I threw up all over the inside of our new car. I stumbled from the car and then threw up on the lawn. Chris took out the garden hose and washed down the yard.

By morning my vomiting had finally stopped. I was exhausted. I felt some cramping and was experiencing stomach-flu-like symptoms. By evening, the cramping was more intense, so I called my doctor—who told me to go the emergency room immediately.

By the time I arrived at the hospital, my contractions were four minutes apart and my cervix had dilated a centimeter. I was only twenty-seven weeks pregnant—most twin pregnancies last about thirty-six weeks.

The nurse set up an IV drip with terbutaline to stop the contractions. The contractions slowed, but when my doctor examined me the next morning, his expression was panicked. One of the twins was ninety percent effaced, meaning there was ninety percent destruction of my uterine cervix. I would have to spend the duration of the pregnancy in the hospital, in bed, with my lower body elevated to prevent pressure on my cervix.

My husband was working twelve hours a day. He had a young son, who was living us and who needed his father, too. I don't know how Chris did it all. He would rush home from work to feed his son, then come to the hospital and hold my hand every night. He took care of everything. It was a special time for us, and we became even closer.

The terbutaline made my heart race and I experienced severe heartburn. After several days, my contractions stopped, and the nurse took me off the IV. I started taking the terbutaline orally, and I was moved out of intensive care. I could get up only to use the restroom. I spent the next several days in bed, my lower body elevated.

I always looked forward to my next meal, and the hospital food was actually quite good. By the twenty-ninth week, I looked like a beached whale. I was enormous. But it didn't matter. Every day I kept the pregnancy going increased the chances of my twins' survival.

After spending eighteen days in bed, my mood darkened. I grew irritable. The heartburn would not let up, and I was developing painful bedsores. I missed being single. I feared that the pregnancy was a mistake. I decided my biological clock had played a mean trick on me, making me believe I wanted to be a mother. I was clueless about motherhood. I had never even changed a diaper.

The next night, the contractions returned. I called the nurse. It was evident that I was in labor again. She set up an IV drip. The terbutaline was no longer working, and the nurse switched the medicine to magnesium. But by the next night, the contractions had grown more intense.

I never had a chance to take a Lamaze class to prepare me for childbirth—all I knew was that Lamaze had something to do with breathing. Chris spent the night at the hospital by my side. He stayed awake all night and felt every contraction with me.

The Birth
It was Friday morning, and I had been in labor thirty-two hours. My doctor arrived shortly after 8 a.m. He examined me and discovered

that I was four and a half centimeters dilated and one of the twins was breeched—in other words, the hind end of the body would emerge first. He said he would have to perform an emergency Cesarean section, and he left the room to prepare for surgery.

Chris came to my bed and held me as we both wept. I was only thirty weeks pregnant.

I was wheeled into surgery around 9 a.m. The anesthesiologist prepared me for a spinal block. My doctor and his colleague came in to deliver the twins. Two more doctors came in from the neonatal intensive care unit (NICU); each of the four doctors had a nurse to assist him. Including my husband and me, twelve people were in the delivery room.

Everything seemed surreal, though the mood was relaxed. I felt no pain as the doctor made the incision. At 9:20 the first twin was delivered. My husband cried. He cut the umbilical cord. We named our firstborn Erik. He weighed three pounds and two ounces, a good weight, I was told, considering how premature he was. Doctors use the Apgar scale to determine a newborn's level of health of a baby. Ten is the highest score. At birth, Erik's score was eight; five minutes later he was upgraded to nine. Before the nurse took Erik to the NICU, she paused briefly so I could kiss him on the forehead.

Chris was full of emotion as the doctors struggled to deliver the second twin, who put up a good fight. The mood changed, and there was no time for my husband to cut the umbilical cord. The baby was dark blue and had to be rushed to the NICU. I didn't even get a glimpse of him. His Apgar score was four, though five minutes later it was upgraded to a nine. I was told he weighed three pounds and four ounces. We named him Westley.

I don't recall leaving the delivery room. I woke up, disoriented, in the recovery room. The doctor from the NICU paid me a visit. He told me the first twin was doing better than expected; however, Westley had challenges. His lungs were underdeveloped, resulting in hyaline membrane disease. The next forty-eight hours were critical. Both the boys were in incubators.

I felt fatigued and too ill to see my babies. After a bedridden three weeks, I began to develop pneumonia. Chris brought me a Polaroid picture of the boys. I never let that photo out of my eyesight.

I was unable to visit the NICU until the third day. I held Erik first.

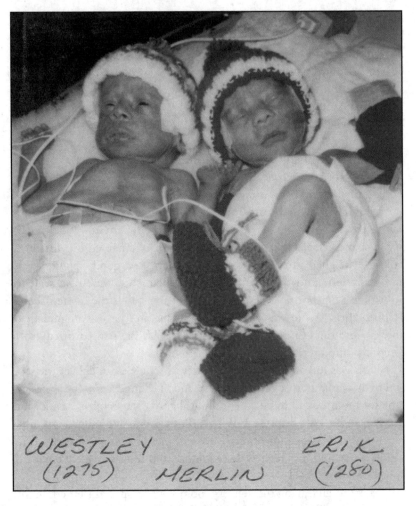

WESTLEY
(1275)   MERLIN   ERIK
                              (1280)

Westley and Erik in NICU. Notice Westley's sunken chest.

He was tiny. He opened his eyes and looked right at me. I knew he couldn't actually see me, but my heart swelled with love.

The NICU was a busy and noisy place. I wanted to be alone to bond with my babies. I knew the nurses were observing me, and it made me feel uncomfortable. I gave Erik back to the nurse and walked to Westley's incubator. He was hooked up to a ventilator, with several wires attached to him. His underdeveloped lungs had caused his chest to appear caved in. I watched him for a few minutes and returned to my room to cry. If only I could have carried the pregnancy a few more weeks. I felt like a failure.

The boys would have to stay in the NICU for several weeks so they could develop a sucking reflex to take in enough fluids and gain weight. I felt strange leaving the hospital without them. I would visit them every day. I had to pump milk from my breasts every three hours, to supply them with nourishment. Fortunately my milk supply was abundant.

When the boys were three weeks old, the doctor told us Westley had developed a staph infection and meningitis, and Erik had bleeding from his rectum. And there was more bad news: the doctor warned Erik might have necrotizing enterocolitis, a fatal disease that destroys all or part of the baby's bowel.

Both babies were started on antibiotics. The staff said someone would call us if the twins took a turn for the worse.

The phone rang at two in the morning. My heart raced. I thought the nurses were calling to say both boys had died. My husband answered the phone. It was his sister; she wanted us to know that she had admitted my mother-in-law to the hospital that night. Needless to say we were concerned but relieved; still, I could not go back to sleep. The next day the boys were improving, and we learned that Erik didn't have necrotizing enterocolitis after all.

At seven weeks Erik was ready to go home. He weighed a whopping five pounds—he hadn't been due to be born for three more weeks. He cried every two hours to be fed. I was exhausted and could not imagine having another baby to take care of.

Westley had to remain on the ventilator for one month after his birth. Once he was removed from the ventilator, he was put on oxygen for the next two and a half months. I took Erik with me every day to visit Westley, who, at that point, was described by the hospital as a "failure to thrive." He had difficulty sucking from his bottle. The nurses would heat my breast milk so I could feed him, and it took what seemed like forever to get any substantial amount of milk into him. Westley remained withdrawn, and I struggled to bond with him. I watched all the other preemies go home as he remained behind. I was tired of going to the NICU every day, yet I could not bring him home the way he was.

Going Home

After three and a half months, Westley no longer required oxygen; however, he was still a slow feeder. The doctors gave him steroid injections, and he slowly improved. At four months the doctors decided he was ready to go home. He weighed seven and a half pounds and could only take in sixteen ounces of milk a day. A doctor warned us either he would sink or swim.

Westley was sent home wearing an apnea monitor, a device for observing heart function. At home he took less and less milk as the days passed. He wouldn't wake up to be fed and refused to take a bottle when I woke him. By the eighth day he was taking in just eight ounces of milk every twenty-four hours. I took him to the pediatrician, and Westley was readmitted to the hospital.

Westley had an enlarged liver—hepatomegaly—because of fluid retention, and he was given an injection of a diuretic called Lasix (generically known as furosemide), as well as other diuretic medicines. He returned from the hospital after a few days, still on diuretics. He remained withdrawn, made little eye contact, and cried when I held him. It was evident that we would need help with Westley. We were at a loss, and the social worker at the hospital suggested that we hire a nurse to feed him at night.

The nurse arrived regularly at 8 p.m. and inserted a gavage feeding tube into Westley's nose, passed it down into his stomach, and fed him. It wasn't easy: Westley screamed and arched his back and sometimes made it impossible to insert the tube. Before long he had to be readmitted to the hospital for another Lasix shot. He remained in the hospital for three days.

Two weeks later I returned to work. I had no choice. We needed the double insurance coverage. My insurance company covered what the primary insurance didn't. A babysitter came to the house during the day and did the best she could. Usually it took forty-five minutes to feed Westley two ounces of milk, and then he often threw it up. He just wanted to stay in his swing and suck his pacifier.

Meanwhile, Erik was proving to be an easy baby. He was friendly and invariably smiling. He was progressing and gaining weight. Westley, on the other hand, was distant and cranky. He still often cried when we held him. Even though he remained a slow feeder, I felt reassured that the gavage feedings at night helped him. But one evening, the nurse again had trouble inserting the feeding tube, and Westley went back to the hospital for the third time. His liver had become enlarged again, and he needed another Lasix shot.

I went straight from work to the hospital to visit him, and one of the doctors came down from the NICU to pay me a visit. He seemed upset—with me. He told me the hospital was doing the same things the nurses at our house were doing, and the problem was mine: we needed family counseling. I knew the doctor was wrong, but I was too emotionally exhausted to argue, so I remained silent.

Westley came back home, and it remained pretty much the same story. He would do okay for a few days, then slide back downhill. He was rigid and did not want to be held.

A nurse came to the house one evening at 8 and tried to insert the feeding tube. Again and again, Westley arched his back and screamed, and the nurse couldn't insert the tube. She called another nurse for assistance—who couldn't insert the tube, either. They called the supervising nurse, and she was unsuccessful as well. By 11 p.m., Westley had been screaming for three hours. My husband asked the nurses to stop trying and sent them home. I admitted him to the hospital for the fourth time.

The following day I left work early to visit Westley. I kept remembering what the doctor from the NICU had said to me. I was hurt and angry. By the time I arrived at the hospital, I was defensive. As I approached Westley's room, I heard him screaming. I walked in his room, and the nurse looked frantic. She could not insert the feeding tube. She looked up at me and asked, "How do you do it?" I told her the nurses coming to our house were having the same problem. She took a business card out of her pocket and handed it to me. "Call this nurse," she said. "She specializes in high-risk infant care. Her name is Junelle Pearson."

After Westley was released from the hospital, we hired Junelle to take over his case. Junelle could see that we were a family in crisis. She was a smart, warm, supportive person with a positive attitude. When Westley cried, she rocked him, holding him in a fetal position. He was rigid. Westley had been so premature, Junelle explained, that he "missed" being curled up in the womb, where developmental fine-tuning takes place. She also noticed that the previous nursing agency was using an adult-size gavage tube, which was trapping air in his stomach. That mistake ex-

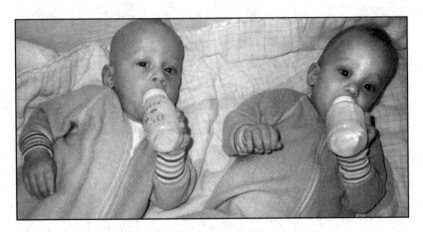

Westley and Erik at twelve months.

plained his crankiness and why he fought so hard against the gavage tube. Fortunately, Junelle came with a supply of infant-size gavage tubes. The next morning Westley woke up smiling.

I had a good feeling about Junelle. She could feel when his liver was enlarged so we could take him to the pediatrician's office for a Lasix shot, which prevented him from being hospitalized again.

Every night Junelle held Westley in a fetal position, and she rocked him for several minutes as he cried. She bent his legs and arms to loosen him up. In about a week he was no longer sobbing when we held him, and shortly after that he was crying to be held. We could finally bond. It was hard enough dealing with his physical health, but I was equally concerned about his emotional development. At about eight months he began to emerge from his shell. Not only did he make great eye contact, but he also looked as if he was looking right into my soul. There was something deep about this baby.

Junelle often discussed early intervention with us. She said premature infants are at high risk for being delayed, and they need to be enrolled in infant/toddler programs to help them with their development. Because of my babies' low birth weights, their risk of becoming developmentally disabled, and Westley's hyaline membrane disease, they qualified for state funding from the Department of Developmental Services. Services are provided through state-operated developmental centers and contracts with non-profit agencies called regional centers. A caseworker from the

Westside Regional Center came to our house to evaluate the kids and suggested services that would benefit them.

Chris and I were excited by the boys' developmental improvements. Even though Erik was premature, he was crawling, sitting up, and walking by the time he turned one. When Westley's swing stopped rocking, his brother pushed the swing again. They had a special bond.

Westley continued to need an occasional Lasix shot for water retention, as well as his other diuretic medicines. Nonetheless, we were thrilled with the progress he had made. Not all was well, however: during an appointment at the pediatrician's office, the doctor noticed Westley's stiffness and told us he was at high risk for developing cerebral palsy. It was a prediction I could not accept. I automatically went into denial. (Luckily, his prediction turned out not to be true: two and a half years later, a pediatrician would rule out cerebral palsy.)

Junelle continued to work with Westley by helping him roll over and push himself up. She was relentless in talking to us about early intervention, even though many doctors adopt the "let's wait and see" philosophy because they don't want to alarm the parents unnecessarily. Yet the first three years of life can have the greatest impact on development. The brain is ninety percent developed by the time a child turns three.

Junelle was vindicated when the *Los Angeles Times* ran a front-page article titled "Early Help Cuts Premature Babies' Risks, Study Finds." The article reported that 250,000 babies are born underweight in the United States each year. Those children who received medical and family support as well as early education enjoyed significant increases in their developmental potential and quality of life. The nationwide study of 985 premature low-birth-weight babies found that those enrolled in an early education program in the first three years of life scored up to thirteen points higher than others on IQ tests and were half as likely to develop behavioral problems.

As a new mother, I had no children to compare my children with—except each other. Erik and Westley had such different personalities. Erik was the party boy, always smiling, playful, and inquisitive. Westley was the serious one. He seemed to be the thinker—even though I frequently observed Westley banging his head against the back of his highchair while he ate his meals. They both talked in their own language that nobody could understand. I was told that twins often create a language of their own and that it was not unusual for preemies to have speech delays. I assumed the boys would catch up sooner, rather than later.

Westley started to take his first steps at fourteen and a half months. He was clumsy and had a tendency to fall and bump into things. One day while we were outside on the patio, he fell, smashed his forehead, and developed an egg-size bump. I cried harder than Westley. I kept ice on it as much as he would allow me to. Not long after that episode, he fell and received a bad cut above his eyelid. It needed seven stitches.

At Junelle's urging I took him to UCLA to be evaluated by Dr. Judy Howard. She observed Westley for several minutes, turned to me, then said, "What a fascinating child." She found him stubborn, controlling, and intelligent. It was her sense that he was quite bright, and because he'd been sick for so long, he developed head banging as a way to soothe himself. She did not observe any autistic-like features or mental retardation and recommended a preschool toddler program once he turned eighteen months old.

Dr. Howard also evaluated Erik and concluded that his physical and neurological exams were normal. His rate of development was average or above average for a toddler who'd been born pre-term, though he had some fine motor skill delays in how he used his hands to work with puzzles. Erik was easygoing and delightful, Dr. Howard said, and he would also benefit from a toddler preschool.

The boys continued to talk in their shared language. I occasionally discerned a recognizable word, such as "dog" or "ball." When Erik was eighteen months old, I heard him say, "Bye-bye, Dada" as my husband pulled out of the driveway. I was thrilled.

One day, the boys' aunt came by and gave them a puzzle, designated for ages three to five. I thanked her but explained the children wouldn't be able to put together a puzzle that advanced. Erik promptly dumped all the pieces out and completed it in seconds.

Erik was quite a climber, too, and it wasn't long before he was climbing out of his crib. I was concerned that his brother would try to copy him.

Westley was beginning to thrive, and it appeared that the medical crisis was over. It was time to say good-bye to Junelle. My husband and I were grateful to her, for she saved all of us from a crisis on many levels. One of the greatest gifts she gave was her belief in me. I was strong, she told me, and a good mother. It was challenging enough being a mother

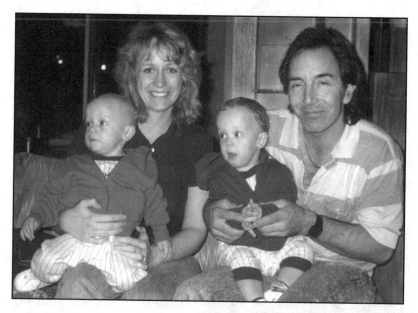

Deborah and Chris, with Westley (left) and Erik at Eighteen months.

with twins. Having twins with special needs put motherhood on a whole other level. We needed all the help and encouragement we could get. Junelle was heaven-sent. If not for her, my kids could have easily fallen through the cracks.

Addressing their needs had proven costly. Thankfully, we had insurance. In adding up all the medical costs for Westley in his first eighteen months of life, we arrived at a figure of about $450,000. That included the NICU, four hospitalizations, and in-home nursing. Erik's tab from the NICU was around $85,000.

The Terrible Twos

When the boys were twenty-seven months old, I stopped working and stayed at home to care for them. Westley was thriving, and double insurance was no longer a necessity. Even though their language was delayed, they certainly knew their numbers and letters, thanks to a heavy dosage of *Sesame Street*. Erik could identify numbers up to twenty-five.

Naptime was always a challenge. One afternoon I put the boys down for a nap. About fifteen minutes later I heard laughter coming from their

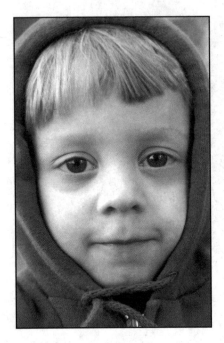

Erik at two years.

room. I opened the door. Erik had taken off all his clothes. Westley was standing on his bookcase with his diapers off, pulling his shirt over his head, ready to fall and hit his head again. They had ripped all the pages out of their Little Golden Books. I was in for a double dosage of the terrible twos.

Erik loved *National Geographic*. The living room floor was always covered with magazines. He pulled them out of the living room bookcase and opened them to the elephant pictures. Later, Erik developed a new fascination: dinosaurs. When he spoke, I couldn't understand him—but I knew he was talking about dinosaurs.

I took the boys to be evaluated at the Westside Regional Center. I knew they had language delays; however, I was surprised to learn that Westley's language skills were at a fourteen-and-a-half-month level. His social skills were at a twelve-and-a-half-month level. He was more than one year delayed. His fine motor, gross motor, and cognitive skills were eight months behind. Erik's language skills were at a fourteen-and-a-half-month level. His social skills were at a twenty-month level. His fine motor, gross motor, and cognitive skills were six months delayed.

At last I comprehended the importance of early intervention. Both boys began receiving weekly occupational therapy. They were also placed in an infant/toddler program for children at risk. It was a new program, and they were the first to be enrolled. They attended three days a week for three hours. When they began the program, they were not saying their own names. By the end of the first week, they were not only saying their own names, but also each other's, though they continued to use their own private language.

The downside of the boys being in the toddler program classroom was that they caught frequent infections. Erik had an ongoing ear infection, while Westley had frequent sinus and ear infections. Shortly after they turned two and a half they were on the antibiotic merry-go-round.

Infections aside, the boys made good progress in the toddler program, even though they continued to show global developmental delays. They were described as having difficulties in organization and behavior, particularly in distractibility and impulsivity, and poor registration and modulation of sensory input from their environment. They both had difficulties with oral motor control and fine motor skills.

I began hearing the professionals who worked with my children describe them with an unfamiliar diagnosis: Pervasive Developmental Disorder. At the time I was clueless as to what it meant. I thought it was a professional term for being delayed. I later learned it was another term for autism. The teacher later told me she thought they were both autistic when they began her program. Autistic or not, by the time the boys turned three, they were showing signs of attention deficit hyperactivity disorder (ADHD): distractibility, short attention span, and restlessness.

Preschool

Once the boys turned three, they no longer qualified for Regional Center state funding. It was time for the Los Angeles Unified School District to provide services for them. The Los Angeles Unified School District covered occupational therapy as well as an early education program.

The boys were enrolled in a special educational program with a small student population, one teacher, and an aide. The autistic label followed Erik because he was less interactive than his brother. He continued to speak in his own language and was withdrawn. He knew his numbers, letters, and colors; nevertheless, his vocabulary consisted of about twenty-five words. He continued to obsess about dinosaurs.

Westley also exhibited severe difficulties in receptive and expressive language. His words were unintelligible. I requested that the twins be placed in a classroom that was more language based. At three and a half years old, they were enrolled in an aphasia class. The class was small and taught by a speech therapist and an aide. The classroom consisted of children with significant language delays and high-functioning autism.

Erik's limited attention span and difficulty following directions con-

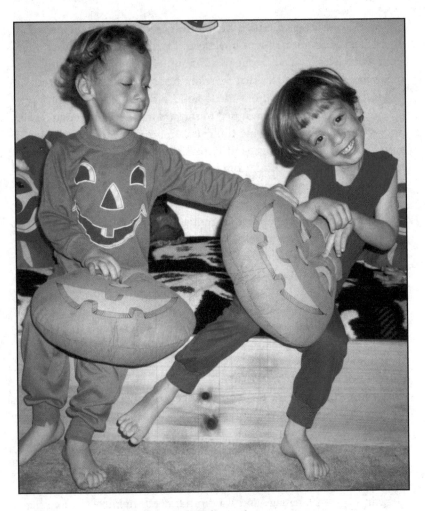

Westley and Erik at three years.

tinued to be a challenge, though he made progress in other areas. He played obsessively with dinosaurs, but he was beginning to make more eye contact with his teachers and his peers.

Westley needed more help with his speech. He had low muscle tone, and his speaking was slushy. While Erik had his dinosaurs, Westley showed unusual preoccupations with his shadow and looking at himself in the mirror. Both boys were described as spacing out at times and had difficulties staying on task. They continued to show poor muscle coordination and poor motor planning in activities. Fine motor skills remained elusive for both boys.

Because Erik was withdrawn and preoccupied with dinosaurs, we were advised to have him evaluated at Regional Center for Autism when he turned four. Our case manager's instinct was that Erik probably didn't have autism, but it would be a good idea to have him evaluated to rule it out. While Westley was a bit on the eccentric side, no one felt that he was showing signs of autism, and he wasn't evaluated.

One month before Erik's fourth birthday I took him to the Regional Center for his assessment. He lined up cars and dolls, a sign of autism. But he made eye contact with the examiner and used up to four words in a sentence. Her findings were that he was not autistic. She noted some distractibility and that he was immature for his age.

We had a pony birthday party for the boys to celebrate their fourth birthday. Usually the boys were friendly and active when we had friends over. This time Erik was unusually withdrawn; he'd go to a corner to play by himself. I was beginning to wonder whether this was the autistic behavior that his teachers were referring to. As it turned out he had an ear infection brewing and did not feel well. He became more social after being on antibiotics for a few days.

The boys were evaluated by their occupational therapist, who concluded that their occupational therapy should be increased to two times a week. They were given the Peabody Development Test, which evaluated their fine motor skills. Westley was more than two years delayed.

When Westley was retested at four and a half years old, it was discovered that his motor skills were at a twenty-five-month level. He had insufficient strength to put interlocking blocks together. He was unable to write his first name and was always the last one to complete a task. He was described as sometimes being in a "dreamlike state."

Erik's fine motor skills were at a thirty-one-month level. He could not cut with scissors. A few isolated skills were tested at a forty-eight-month level. Erik knew numbers up to fifty. Meanwhile, he continued to talk nonstop about dinosaurs.

I dreaded taking the boys to the market with me. They fought over who would sit in the cart seat. It was too intense to take them out. Westley liked to go to the cereal aisle, and Erik searched for dinosaur toys.

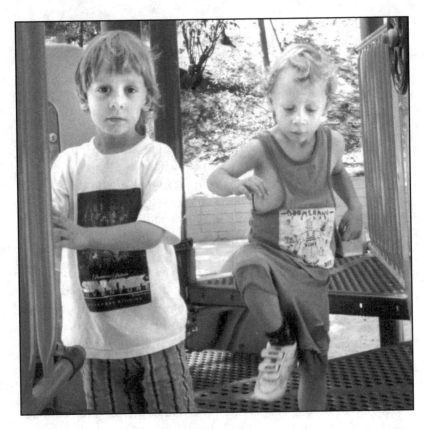

Erik and Westley at three years.

Wherever we went we were noticed because of the boys' high energy level. Usually people would be more accepting of them, once they realized they were twins.

The boys and I had repeated respiratory infections. Erik and Westley visited the pediatrician at least once a month. We were all developing allergies to some of the antibiotics. I had a permanent ear or respiratory infection. My energy was low. I used to attend an aerobics class, but now I could barely complete four minutes on a stationary bicycle.

At about this time, Chris and I decided to move to a new house, right behind a good elementary school. While we were packing up the house, we moved our bed away from the wall—and discovered black mold growing everywhere. I wondered whether it had been behind our chronic infections. I was glad we were moving.

The boys were excited about the new house. Chris and I were, too: it was our hope that Erik and Westley would be able to attend a regular classroom at the neighborhood school by first grade. They were still more than a year away from starting kindergarten.

In the new house I tried to keep the boys busy while I unpacked. I brought their little table and chair into my room and told Erik to draw some pictures. A few minutes later I suggested that he write the alphabet. He replied, "I just did." I was surprised that I could read every letter. Erik's fine motor skills were catching up.

The boys went outside to play on the back porch. I heard them talking through the wall. "Hey, Westley!" Erik said. "Don't tell Mom, but look at what I'm doing." I stopped unpacking and went to see what Erik did not want me to see. He had dumped dirt and small rocks into his play workbench sink. It was a mess. I asked him not to bring dirt and rocks up to the porch. He replied in a matter-of-fact voice, "Those are dinosaur fossils, Mom." At moments like these, Erik reminded me of Dennis the Menace.

Before he got out of bed in the morning, we could hear him loudly lecturing, "The triceratops lived 100 million years ago." I found it interesting to observe a boy who, despite a significant expressive language delay, became so articulate when identifying all the dinosaurs and the facts relevant to them.

Although they could both be charming children, they were also at times difficult. Westley was throwing tantrums, and they were both rebellious. At four and a half, they appeared stuck in the terrible twos. It was time for me to find them professional help.

I found a psychologist who worked with children with behavioral problems. I told her that I thought both boys exhibited ADHD symptoms and that some professionals had found evidence of high-functioning autism, particularly in Erik's case. He was still obsessed with dinosaurs and often acted as though he was not hearing what people said to him. But I made it quite clear that I did not believe that my kids were autistic.

In evaluating Erik, the psychologist found him to be delayed over all by six months. His strengths: blocking, drawing, colors, numbers, body

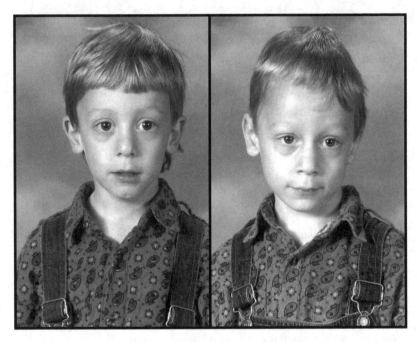

Erik and Westley in preschool.

image, and matching. His weaknesses: fine and gross motor skills, auditory memory, expressive and receptive language, play, and social skills. His spontaneous language often consisted of engaging the examiner in, unsurprisingly, a conversation about dinosaurs. He also sometimes acted as though he did not hear the examiner's requests; he isolated himself from her and continued to play with his dinosaurs. When she examined the boys playing together with their toys, Erik did not interact with his brother.

In evaluating Westley, the psychologist determined he was overall a year delayed. Color labeling, number concepts, and matching were among his strengths; his weaknesses were in the areas of drawing, body image, visual memory, expressive language, play, social development, and gross motor skills. He also exhibited difficulty paying attention and poor impulse control. Westley became frustrated when he could not do a simple task and then threw tantrums. His behavior was becoming aggressive, and he had quite a temper. He flung his toys and hit his brother—yet when he wanted to, Westley could be a charming child.

The psychologist was helpful in her suggestions about disciplining them. We began to create "reward charts" at the end of the day. When the boys earned enough stickers they would receive a small toy. I also began implementing timeouts, which proved more effective with Westley than Erik. Erik could be very belligerent: every time I took the boys out, Erik would demand that I buy him a toy. When I refused, he would throw a tantrum. Westley, on the other hand, rarely asked me to buy him anything.

The boys continued in their aphasia class and were making good progress; however, we were still coming down with frequent respiratory infections and taking antibiotics.

We lived across the street from a small park with playground equipment for young children. The park provided a great opportunity for the boys, now five years old, to work on their gross motor skills. But Westley became frustrated with his lack of coordination. He tended to be accident prone. He watched children much younger than himself climb the circle bars, while he could barely climb them at all.

Meanwhile, Erik was becoming more social. He would seek out new playmates every time we went to the park and was becoming a real boy's boy. Erik had a strong curiosity and enjoyed exploring. He was beginning to speak more appropriately for his age. He continued to obsess on dinosaurs—and developed a new preoccupation: Legos.

Westley was very serious and would usually like to be in the backyard. He played mostly with his stuffed animals and toy telephones and would often have conversations with an imaginary friend.

The one thing I knew for sure is that I did not have run-of-the-mill kids.

When they turned five and a half, I had the boys reevaluated by the psychologist. She reported that Erik continued to use his own language to initiate interactions with others. He made repeated statements, and she said his voice was unusual, distinguished by a mildly hollow tone. But he was making progress and was only seven months delayed overall. She did not come out and say that Erik was autistic; however, she hinted at it. Almost all the professionals who worked with him reported some autistic symptoms. I thought that if he were autistic he would always show the symptoms. The only time I would observe autistic behaviors—

such as being withdrawn and aloof—was when he was coming down with an infection. I suspected that many of the professionals thought I was in denial, that I would not be able to face the truth: that both of my sons were autistic.

In evaluating Westley, the psychologist found him to be very charming and engaging. He had made great progress in some areas, such as auditory memory. Like Erik, he used his own language to initiate conversations. His language was both delayed and idiosyncratic. He also had a lateral lisp. The psychologist suggested that Ritalin could help Westley focus on tasks and materials, sustain both visual and auditory attention, and screen out exogenous stimuli.

When I told Chris that the psychologist had recommended medication for Westley, he became upset. "No way is he going to be taking Ritalin," Chris declared. I told Chris that I would have Westley examined by a psychiatrist. "Go ahead," he replied, "but my answer will remain the same."

I took Westley to the psychiatrist. He gave me the Conners Teacher Questionnaire, enumerating the different symptoms of ADHD as a checklist to be filled out by his teacher. She checked off a slew of symptoms: Westley was restless in a "squirmy" sense, had a short attention span, and was excitable and impulsive much of the time. The teacher hoped he would go on Ritalin. So did the psychiatrist. At this point, a psychologist, a psychiatrist, and a teacher had concluded Westley should be medicated—but my husband was resolute. "Perhaps some children do need it," he said, "but it would not help Westley."

At the Individualized Education Program meeting the teachers recommended that Westley remain in the aphasia class. Due to the boys' gross motor skill delays, they were enrolled in an adaptive physical education course, geared toward children whose gross motor skills were behind and for those with disabilities. The boys continued to receive occupational therapy in school and once a week in the clinic.

Erik's gross motor skills remained about one year behind. He was making very good progress in other areas. By the time he was five and a half his fine motor skills were at age level. He continued to fixate on dinosaurs, in addition to a new interest—the color red. He was described as having a good self-image and was making progress in his social skills. The major concern was that he liked to tease other children and test limits in the classroom rules. At the Individualized Education Program meeting the teachers recommended for the next year that Erik be mainstreamed into a regular kindergarten class for two and a half hours and then return to the aphasia class for speech therapy.

Kindergarten

I was a little nervous and excited about Erik being mainstreamed into kindergarten. He was going from a small class to an overcrowded one. His attention disorder presented a challenge for the teacher, and his disruptive behavior persisted.

One day Erik came home from school with a distressing note from his teacher. The kindergarten class had worked hard in recycling cans and paper, earning enough money to buy good scissors for the classroom. Erik destroyed the scissors by covering them with glue. The teacher was unable to remove the glue and sent us the scissors in a bag, so we could see them.

I decided I should go and observe Erik in school so I could see what was going on firsthand. I arrived at his class while the children were at recess. When they returned, Erik walked right pass me—he didn't notice I was in the classroom. All the children sat down, and Erik was in the back. While the teacher was talking, Erik flipped through big pictures hanging on the easel. The teacher twice asked him to stop.

I knew Erik was a handful for his teacher. I could see the stress on her face in dealing with him. He always required adult supervision to get back on task. I felt guilty and frustrated about the situation. And I really felt bad for the teacher.

Meanwhile, Westley was making good academic progress. His reading, math, and spelling skills were at age level. He was described as being friendly, and he got along well with his peers. His two favorite things to do during free time at school were to play house in the little house in the schoolyard and dress up in costumes. Unfortunately, his fine and gross motor skills remained delayed, and his attention disorder was an ongoing issue. He frequently looked in the mirror at his reflection or watched his shadow.

When the boys turned six, I had them reevaluated by the psychologist. Erik was given the Peabody Individual Achievement Test, which indicated that he'd made great progress in many areas and was demonstrating beginning-to-mid-kindergarten level capabilities. His most significant areas of weakness continued to be in behavior, language, and gross motor skills. The psychologist noted that he was wiggly and fidgety and, at times, would not remain seated. She said he had symptoms of ADHD. The psychologist recommended that Erik be mainstreamed in a regular first grade class in the coming year, with speech-language therapy and adaptive physical education to help him meet his gross motor skills delays. Finally, she used the M-word—she suggested medicine to target his distractibility and hyperactive behaviors.

Westley's evaluation was much more alarming. He had made little progress since the last test. His greatest strengths were in body image, auditory memory, and number skills. His areas of weaknesses included fine motor, gross motor, and puzzle skills, as well as sustained attention to tasks, strategy development, and frustration tolerance. Overall, Westley was delayed by eighteen months.

The psychologist went on to say that Westley exhibited a complex fantasy life. He had brought a stuffed animal with him, which he put down for a nap during the session. After the testing, he related to the psychologist a dream that he said the stuffed animal had while they were working. The dream involved his family members and the circus. She found this behavior to be odd. He repeatedly asked her where Erik and I went during the testing, even though he knew the answer. She recommended that Westley continue in the aphasia class for the following year, with occupational therapy and adaptive physical education—and that, like Erik, he should be considered for a medicine trial.

I knew it was going to be futile to discuss the medication issue with Chris. He strongly opposed Ritalin. I had mixed feelings about it. In doing research, I discovered that Ritalin (generically known as methylphenidate) suppressed appetite and growth—and my kids were already only between the tenth and twenty-fifth percentile for their height and weight. I also learned that some of the side effects of Ritalin were motor tics and a set of behaviors comparable to Tourette's syndrome. Westley already had recurring facial tics, and I worried that Ritalin may possibly exacerbate his Tourette's-like behaviors. And I was confused why doctors were recommending Ritalin when they knew that Westley had facial tics.

The kids had been through enough because of their premature birth. They were both bright, and it was my husband's gut feeling that they would both be okay without taking drugs. On the other hand, it was me who was with them most of the time. Raising twins with an attention disorder was stressful to the point that it had an impact on my health. I was always sick with ear infections, bronchitis, headaches, and chronic fatigue. I felt pressure from teachers always complaining about my kids' hyperactivity.

The psychologist could not understand Chris' aversion to Ritalin: it had been around forever, and millions of children were taking it. "Just try it for a few weeks and see if you see an improvement," she said. Chris told me to get a second opinion.

I took them to another psychiatrist. It had been raining hard. The boys were more hyper than usual. We were on the second floor, on our way to the doctor's office, when Erik disappeared. All of the sudden I heard screaming and crying echoing throughout the courtyard. He was lying on the ground outside. I thought he had fallen from the second floor. He had actually walked down the stairs and slipped. He was fine. I was not. I was ready to put them on Ritalin.

The psychiatrist strongly suggested that Erik needed medication. In observing Westley she saw some hints of Tourette's as well as an attention deficit.

I knew Chris would still object to medication. I insisted that he have a private session with the psychiatrist to discuss it. I was hoping she would be able to get through to him.

When Chris came home that night, the first words out of his mouth were: "They are not going to take Ritalin. And if you put them on it, I will divorce you."

"What do you suggest we do?" I asked.

"You have been looking into alternative medicine," he answered. "Try to treat it naturally."

My mother had been visiting us, and she told me about a book called *Is This Your Child?* by Doris Rapp, MD (Harper Paperbacks, 1991). The book linked allergies to hyperactivity, behavior issues, and learning disabilities. My mother told me that my kids looked allergic. She mentioned that they both had dark circles under their eyes. Certainly, something was wrong: it didn't make sense that the boys and I were fighting one infection after another. We were on antibiotics more often than not. I took them to an allergist.

The allergist noted that both appeared allergic. She observed water in Erik's ears. He had frequent ear infections, nasal congestion, and bronchitis. As it turned out, Erik had severe dust-mite allergy. He also was allergic to mold, cats, several weeds, trees, and grasses.

Westley's examination was more alarming. The allergist detected a wheeze and diagnosed it as asthmatic. He also suffered from frequent sinusitis, ear infections, and headaches. At different times of the year he would frequently blink his eyes and clear his throat. The allergist ordered a scratch prick test. Westley tested positive for allergies to cats and mold.

We bought a HEPA filter for the boys' bedroom to control dust and mold, then put dust covers over their mattresses. They had allergy injections two times a week. It was no picnic taking them for their shots. They would rebel by misbehaving. Erik would frequently leave the waiting room and wander around the hallway, while Westley would switch the light on and off in the waiting room. I found myself constantly apologizing for their behavior. The more patients in the waiting room, the more obnoxious they would be: the boys always loved an audience. After an allergy shot they were supposed to wait twenty to thirty minutes before we left, to make sure they had no reaction to the injection. I always found myself cutting out a few minutes early because of their behavior. I bribed them in the hopes they'd behave—I took them for fast food or bought them a toy. I did just about everything, except put them on Ritalin.

The allergist checked the boys frequently to observe how the allergy injections and other measures were working. Erik still had fluid in his ears. The lack of response frustrated all of us. It seemed as if Erik had a permanent ear infection.

I inquired about alternative medicine. The doctors I had been using were wary of alternative approaches and cautioned me to be very careful.

My first step on the alternative path led me to a chiropractor. In researching alternative medicine, I had learned that an aligned spine allows the nervous system to work optimally and can help the immune system function at a higher level, therefore keeping the body healthy. Dr. Neal Snyder understood and sympathized with my kids' situation. He found several misalignments in their spines, and the boys began receiving regular chiropractic treatments.

Meanwhile, my energy level was totally depleted. I was a full-time, stay-at-home mother, and I was too exhausted to volunteer at my kids' school. As soon as they left for school, I would go right back to bed and nurse an ear infection, bronchitis, or a headache. I was also experiencing vertigo.

The boys continued to be out of control when I took them for their allergy shots. After six months of chasing them around the doctor's office and always trying to explain why my kids acted the way they did, I gave up. I had no more energy. I did not care what people thought anymore. I was sure it was obvious that my children had special needs; so be it.

We also had many wonderful moments with our kids. When I took the boys to the park one day, a mother came up to me—to praise Erik. Erik had noticed her daughter crying; he then sat down next to the little girl, put his arm around her, and told her it was okay and that he would share his toys with her. I wish all the professionals who thought he was autistic could have witnessed that moment.

The boys were very affectionate and often played well together. Westley loved dressing up in his old Halloween costumes and playing make-believe. One day he would be Peter Pan and the next, a Power Ranger. He loved Michael Jackson's music and wanted to dance like him. It was a great challenge, thanks to his poor gross motor skills. He would become especially frustrated while attempting the moonwalk. No matter how many times he tried to get the movements down, he couldn't do it.

First Grade

The school bus picked up Westley every day to take him to his new school. A speech pathologist and an assistant taught his aphasia class. His teacher was quite an inspiration to Westley. When he came home from school he would drag a small table from the living room into his bedroom and pretend to be a teacher. He wrote down all his imaginary pupils' names and put grades on their papers. In the course of his playing he managed to complete his homework. In no time he was performing academically at age, or above age, level, though his gross and fine motor skills remained delayed.

Erik attended the elementary school behind our house. He was mainstreamed into a regular first grade with twenty-nine students. Two-thirds of the students were boys. Academically he was performing from average to above for his age. Erik made friends easily and became popular

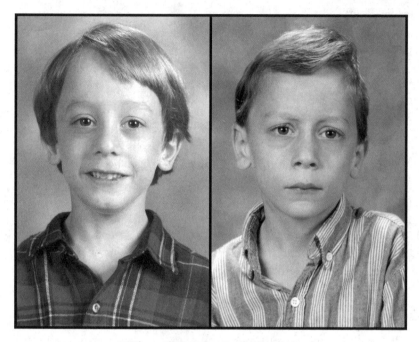

Erik and Westley in first grade.

with the boys' clique. Unfortunately, his teacher found his nonstop talking to be a problem. He lacked verbal self-control and often jumped out of his seat.

His obsession with dinosaurs persisted—he often played with the variety of Transformer toys that metamorphosed into dinosaurs. His interest would make its way into his school work: when the teacher wrote a phrase about Franklin and Eleanor Roosevelt on the chalkboard and asked students to respond with an appropriate drawing, Erik drew a stegosaurus with an American flag covering half of its body. The drawing showed natural talent and imagination.

Westley's therapist went to observe him at school. She said he was standing in line with the other children when he suddenly started to twitch and jerk his head around, watching his shadow. I laughed; I knew he was doing his impression of Michael Jackson. Unfortunately, he was calling negative attention to himself. The other children would make fun of him, and he would become upset. Westley was a worrier, but also very sensitive and caring. The adults really liked him because he was different and an interesting child to watch. He was often described as walking to the beat of his own drum. Whenever we went into a store he would find a mirror to look at his reflection. This had been going on since he was a toddler.

Erik had good and bad days at school. He needed a lot of help staying on task. When he became too much to handle, the teacher would send him to the other first grade class until he could contain himself. His teacher said that at one point, he was crawling on the floor, imitating a lizard.

After hearing about this, the psychologist couldn't understand why we wouldn't put Erik on Ritalin. I knew I had to do something. I was burned out going to the doctors all the time. Chris was working twelve hours a day, often six days a week. On his one day off, he would be an enormous help; however, it was never enough.

Exhausted, I went to the doctor. I was diagnosed with Hashimoto's thyroiditis, an autoimmune disease causing an under-active thyroid. The diagnosis explained why I was chronically tired. The thyroid medicine helped take the edge off, but I was still tired and had frequent headaches and infections.

We had good insurance coverage; nevertheless, the medical deductibles, along with all of our other medical needs, were taking their toll on our finances. Chris believed that we were spending too much money on doctors and allergy medicines, with little progress. At this point, I decided to look into alternative medicine beyond chiropractic. If my husband wouldn't allow the kids to go on Ritalin, then I would try the alternative path, even though our insurance would not cover most of it.

My chiropractor suggested that I take my kids to see a Traditional Chinese Medical (TCM) doctor. I visited him first to check him out and see if he could really help us. He took me off all dairy products and sugar. He gave me awful-tasting Chinese herbs to take every day. I knew my kids would not put up with the herbs and would resist the dietary restrictions. They loved dairy products, and Erik was addicted to milk.

Regardless, after one month, I began to feel better and the ear infections and vertigo vanished—and I decided it might be worth our while to take the kids to see him. He examined both of them and requested we remove dairy and sugar from their diet. He allowed them one serving of fruit a day. I managed, by some miracle, to get them off dairy, and I reduced their sugar intake as well. I began buying soy milk, though they didn't care for it.

At the Chinese doctor's office, I learned that cow's milk and other dairy products are toxic to humans—cow dairy is designed for calves, not people. More than thirty years of research shows cow dairy to be connected to colic; ear infections; allergies; asthma; chronic sinusitis; menstrual problems; lung, breast, ovarian, and uterine cancer; heart disease; and diabetes in children. Dairy products have antibiotic and pesticide residues, which also damage the immune system. I didn't want to expose my family to any more pesticides, so I began to buy organic produce at the farmer's market.

When Erik's allergist examined him a month later, she noticed that the fluid in his ears had vanished. He was no longer getting ear infections. It appeared that a dairy allergy had been the problem. His teacher and I could see a difference. He still talked too much but was beginning to make a real effort to improve his behavior. Convinced that dairy should be permanently removed from my children's diets, I began to purchase calcium-fortified juices and calcium supplements.

Dairy allergies cost my family countless infections and visits to the doctor's office. Not one of our doctors ever suspected that dairy products were the cause of Erik's or my persistent ear infections. They'd just continued to prescribe antibiotics.

We did not continue to see the Chinese doctor because his office was too far away. He'd gotten us on the right path though, and I was grateful for that. I had many revelations about Erik's autistic symptoms and strongly believed that the chronic fluid in his ears had contributed to his autistic-like behavior.

Erik began to complain profusely about being pulled out of class for adaptive physical education. He wanted to be in regular P.E. with all his buddies. The adaptive P.E. teacher tested Erik and found his gross motor skills were at age level, and he was placed in regular P.E. His speech had also improved, and he was becoming quite articulate.

Chris insisted that it was time for Westley to be mainstreamed for second grade. Academically he was flying. He was a natural speller and received 100 percent on all of his spelling tests. His expressive language had improved, although his speech remained slushy, due to low muscle tone. His vocabulary and reading skills were above age level, and his tic-like movements were diminishing.

He remained somewhat eccentric, and we hoped that being with mainstream children would help him catch up socially. He would need to continue in adaptive P.E., speech therapy, and occupational therapy to address his fine motor skills. Considering everything he had been through, we were very pleased with his progress.

Second Grade

My husband's hunches were correct. Westley made a smooth transition to full inclusion into second grade. He went from a class of eight students to twenty-nine students with one teacher. His academic skills were above average. His handwriting remained very poor. His obsession with Michael Jackson was beginning to fade. *Star Wars* was his new thing—he wanted to be Luke Skywalker.

Erik made good academic progress and remained popular among his peers. The biggest obstacle was his motor mouth. The teacher would leave messages on the answering machine saying that Erik's talking had advanced to a new level. He still had poor impulse control. The only service he was receiving at that time was a full-inclusion teacher. She would visit the classroom once a week to check on his progress and offer suggestions to the teacher.

The school principal said that my boys were the perfect students for full inclusion. They were overly qualified for special education, however, and still had to be monitored to make sure they were making progress. We were fortunate to be receiving so many services.

One day, Westley got into trouble in the schoolyard at lunchtime. He was climbing up on the table with the other boys when a mother who had volunteered for yard duty asked them to get off the table. The boys called her names, and Westley told her she stank. They were brought to the principal's office. The kids stayed after school to write an apology. The teacher said that Westley was truly remorseful and quite shaken by what he had done. He was having a hard time making friends and would hang around the kids who tended to get into mischief. They were the only ones who would accept him.

I continued to have second thoughts about Ritalin. I kept in touch with the psychiatrist who had originally diagnosed Westley with ADHD.

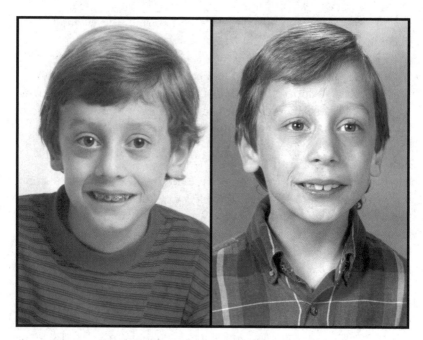

Erik and Westley in second grade.

He said as long as he was making academic progress he would be okay not taking Ritalin.

Adults enjoyed Westley because he was unique, unusually sensitive, and insightful. I was amazed at the questions he would ask me. He asked me whether the universe could move. I was clueless as to how to answer him. I know I wasn't asking those kinds of questions in second grade!

The boys still received allergy shots once a week. Erik was beginning to mature and didn't give me such a hard time. Westley was another story. He was very defiant and would not go to the nurse when it was his turn for a shot. He would scream when he received his injection. Back in the waiting room, he continued to act out. Once we got home and he had calmed down, I would ask him why he would act this way every time he received a shot. His reply would be that he couldn't help it and that he didn't want to go anymore. At times it seemed that Westley really didn't care what people thought of him. Usually he was sweet and engaging, but he was also unpredictable.

When Westley reached the end of the second grade, everyone was pleased with his academic progress, though his teacher said that he remained socially awkward. It was difficult for children and adults to understand him. He was still uncoordinated and would have to remain in adaptive physical education. He continued to have sinus infections, but not as frequently as before.

The boys played well together most of the time, except that Westley would scratch, bite, kick, or hit his brother when he became angry. They were both into *Star Wars* and loved action figures. Westley loved his toys too much—he would chew on them. Concerned about possible lead exposure, I called the toy companies, who assured me that their products were lead-free. Nonetheless, I was constantly asking Westley to get toys out of his mouth.

He also resisted using his utensils at mealtime. I often wondered whether his low muscle tone was preventing him from using a fork or knife. He would finger feed himself all his peas, rice, cereal, meat, and pasta. The only time he'd use a spoon was while eating yogurt. All his books would be smeared with barbeque sauce or whatever he had just eaten.

I was tired of nagging my kids or telling them what they were doing wrong, and I probably let too many things slide in regard to their poor daily habits. I was told to choose my battles wisely. When they did something right, I went overboard praising them. I didn't want them to suffer poor self-esteem.

When the boys were in second grade, the state of California started to use the Stanford 9 Achievement Test for evaluating students' academic skills, identifying where they stood compared to other children their age across the country. The boys' test results were weak in some areas, but overall, they were in the ballpark for the average child. Westley excelled in spelling, where his scores ranked in the eighty-second percentile. Erik was making good progress, with age-appropriate scores in all areas.

Third Grade
The full-inclusion teacher would visit the boys' classrooms once a week to monitor their progress. Westley continued with a full range of services to meet his needs. He had an occupational therapist work with him at school to address his poor handwriting skills. He continued with speech

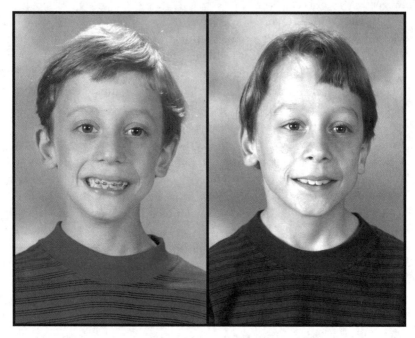

Erik and Westley in third grade.

therapy and adaptive physical education.

Even though Westley was making good academic progress, I saw a regression in his handwriting. It was getting much worse. He was also becoming more aggressive toward Erik. He often scratched, hit, kicked or bit him.

Erik still had some behavioral issues of his own, including poor impulse control. But he was always happy and appeared to have high self-esteem. He had many friends in and out of school and was quite social. Westley, on the other hand, was having a challenging time with other children. He frequently ate lunch alone. Erik told me that he would see his brother walking around in circles and talking to himself. Sometimes it would appear that he was talking to a tree. Kids were beginning to make fun of him. Erik would sometimes ask his brother to join him for lunch, but Westley would decline. He wanted to make his own friends.

Every week we took the boys out to dinner at a restaurant—where Westley generally went out of his way to embarrass us. He would yell or kick his chair. The yelling and poor attitude would begin on the way to the restaurant. Once dinner came, we would all manage to calm down and enjoy our meal. His father would ask him, "Whatever happened to the old Westley?"

I usually refused to be drawn into Westley's dramatic scenes; I felt that by giving him too much attention I would add more fuel to the fire. Instead, we would take privileges away and give him timeouts. It would work for a day or two, but he continued to suffer from a lack of impulse control and often seemed agitated.

School was closed the day before Thanksgiving. I had to take the boys on some errands. First, I went to the Santa Monica Farmer's Market. It was a mob scene, so we went to another market to pick up the turkey. We were standing at the deli when Westley suddenly went ballistic on Erik. He started to strangle him and knocked him on the ground. You could see red fingerprints on Erik's neck. A woman standing at the deli witnessed the whole thing and appeared horrified. I got them out of the market as quickly as possible. On the way home I gave Westley a major tongue-lashing. I told him that when he got home he would spend the rest of the day cleaning his room, and that he did. He found long-lost toys, cleaned out his entire closet, and did an incredible job. Then he wrote his brother an apology.

As the school year progressed, Erik decided that he didn't want to do his homework anymore. He was constantly sneaking away from the table, and I would have to bring him back to task. Westley would rush through his homework, and it was impossible to read his handwriting.

It was an emotionally draining time. We had stopped seeing the psychologist—I was tired of being told to put my kids on Ritalin. And in addition to the challenge the boys presented on a daily basis, both of my husband's parents had passed away within nine months of each other.

When the boys were at the end of third grade, we had their Individualized Education Program meeting. Although it was recommended that Westley continue to receive all the supporting services already in place, the teacher reported he was showing substantial improvements, academically and socially. He was reading at age level, with the more advanced group. He had established some friendships and shown growth in the classroom activities. Everyone felt that Westley had made progress—everyone except for me. I was seeing a decline, not only in his schoolwork, but also socially. We received the results for the Stanford 9 achievement test series. He made great progress in his reading skills, but he dropped significantly in math and language. The most alarming was his spelling score, which had dropped from eighty-second percentile the year before to the twentieth percentile. I believed that he mistakenly checked off the wrong answers—his attention disorder was probably to blame.

Erik's teacher reported that he was at grade level or slightly above. He had a challenging time with organization skills and didn't take his studies seriously. His behavior was somewhat immature and could be triggered by the behavior of others. But overall, the teacher was happy with Erik's progress and recommended that the full-inclusion teacher continue to monitor him in fourth grade.

Fourth Grade
In fourth grade Erik got one of the most popular teachers—who gave relatively little homework. I was pleased, as I also needed a break. I could use a year off from constantly nagging Erik to do his homework. All that was required was one national current-event report each week. His teacher subscribed to the philosophy of teaching kids how to think instead of what to think. Erik continued to face the challenge of staying on task and using self-control. But he was becoming a real history buff and made new friends.

Westley's fourth-grade teacher was perfect for him; her approach was both structured and creative. She was concerned for Westley socially: he had only one friend, and there was an excessive dependency on the friendship that led to many disappointments for him.

Academically, Westley's handwriting continued to be his biggest challenge. Nobody, including Westley, could read it. The occupational therapist would work with him by using a special pencil grip, but it didn't help much. He would rush through his assignments and sneak his work up to the teacher's desk when she was too busy to check it before accepting it. His poor handwriting hurt his math performance. He would not line up his numbers properly and, as a result, could not calculate the correct answer. Yet he was capable of understanding math concepts and had all the multiplication tables memorized.

Westley was also finding an outlet for his imagination and storytelling skills. He loved the creative-writing process, and his teacher saw some true natural talent.

Meanwhile, my health was beginning to improve. I used to go straight back to bed when my kids left for school. Now I was walking three miles every day and loving it. I had enough energy to volunteer at school and teach art history in both of my kids' classes.

Westley, on the other hand, was still experiencing sinus infections and often complained of headaches. He was receiving allergy injections every three weeks. He took a prescription allergy medicine, as well as a nasal spray and an inhaler for his asthma every night before bed. His teacher felt he was having difficulty focusing much of the time. She suspected that he needed to be medicated for an attention disorder.

"Oh, here we go again," I thought. I agreed there was a problem, but Ritalin was not the solution. I explained to her our concerns about Ritalin and added that her suggestion was nothing I hadn't heard many times before. Nothing else was said for a while. Even so, I was again having second thoughts about putting him on a trial run of Ritalin. I was very concerned for Westley—socially, as well as academically. I felt maybe the benefits would outweigh the liabilities of being medicated. I didn't want him to go through life as a failure with low self-esteem. I felt stuck between a rock and a hard place. I dealt with it by not dealing with it. I was burned out and needed a break from constant worry.

But it was hard not to worry about Westley. His teacher told me how the class would play a game to help the students memorize their science facts. When the students couldn't answer the question, she would say, "I am going to give the answer now." Westley would then yell, "Nooooo!" He received A's on some tests and D's on others. If his grade was low, he would become upset and walk around the classroom announcing his grade, saying, "I can't believe I got a D." He would try to calm himself down by telling the students that he was going to be okay. Yet I had never pressured my children to get A's; knowing their challenges, I just wanted them to try their best.

One week, Westley had a sinus infection, which made it difficult to focus. His teacher was concerned, especially after she watched Westley while he thought he was sharpening his pencil in the pencil sharpener—he had neglected to put the pencil in it. His teacher said that he had been totally "spaced out." I felt pretty foolish myself and had no excuse. That night I told my husband about the incident. "No Ritalin," he insisted.

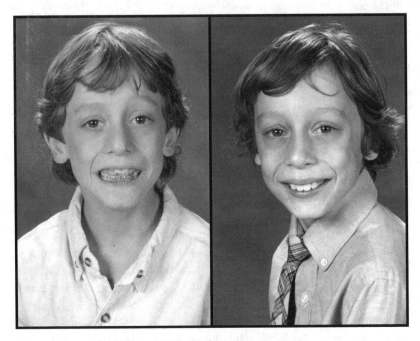

Erik and Westley in fourth grade.

I had recently read research about Ritalin causing cancer in laboratory animals and told Westley's teacher about the article. Her reply was, "Everything causes cancer."

Some people suggested biofeedback. Unfortunately, it was too expensive, and our insurance didn't cover it. I focused on doing what I could afford, especially when it came to what Westley and Erik ate: I visited the Santa Monica Farmer's Market every week to purchase organic fruit and vegetables, and the boys consumed no dairy and very little sugar. I decided to take wheat out of Westley's diet to see if there would be an improvement. He was such a trooper about giving up wheat, but we saw no difference after six weeks.

Meanwhile, Erik was flying academically. His only downfall was physical education. He was too busy socializing to follow the rules or participate enough. But he received mostly A's and loved school, especially his history class. I enjoyed having him tell me about the history I could remember firsthand. He was learning about Vietnam, and I told him how my friends drove from New Jersey to Washington, D.C., to protest against the war in the early 1970's. He asked whether I was a hippie, and I had a good laugh.

The full-inclusion teacher continued to visit both of the boys' classrooms once a week. She was impressed with Westley's sensitivity toward others and his brother. She didn't know how much he attacked Erik at home. Erik would tease him and Westley would react by biting, hitting, kicking or scratching him. Two hours later they would be playing with each other like nothing had happened. I knew most siblings behave in the same manner to varying degrees and assumed this behavior was more common with twins.

At the end of the year we had their Individualized Education Program meeting to discuss the boys' progress. Erik's teacher reported that he excelled academically in every subject and would receive straight A's, though he was still talking too much in the classroom. "Never once did I yell, 'Shut up' to any of the students, until Erik," his teacher sighed. Erik had no other behavior problems, though, and did well socially. It was the consensus of the Individualized Education Program team that all special educational services be discontinued for him.

At Westley's Individualized Education Program meeting the teacher said he had made progress in reading and creative writing. His teacher said that he "gives great details and is able to focus for longer periods of time." His math had improved as well. Science and social studies remained a challenge for him. Socially, he had a problem with interrupting other students. He would continue speech therapy, adaptive physical education, and occupational therapy. Overall he had a C-plus average.

We received the results of the Stanford 9 test over the summer. Erik performed well, except in spelling, where he only scored in the thirty-second percentile. Erik was never a great speller.

Westley's Stanford 9 results were more upsetting—they'd dropped substantially from the previous year. His total reading score was in the fifteenth percentile. His math results had dropped by ten percentile points, and his language score was only in the eighth percentile. The only area he excelled in was spelling, where he scored in the eightieth percentile. Overall, his test scores were far below average.

Why had Westley's scores dropped? He'd been wearing a cast while he was taking the test—I wondered whether it had distracted him. Weeks

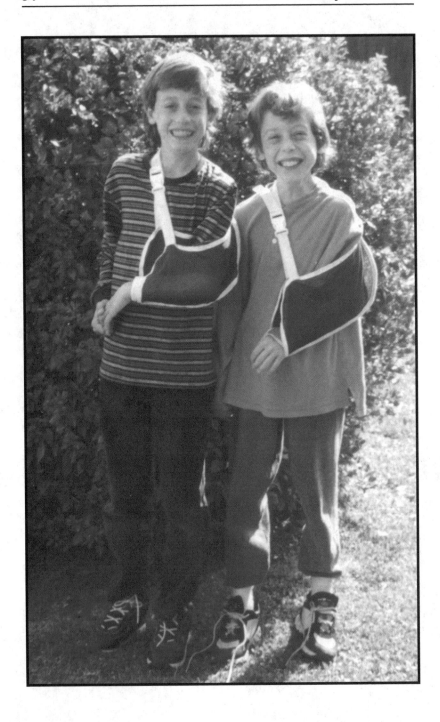

before, he had hurt himself during a game of hide-and-seek. Erik had also injured himself during the game—the boys had managed to fall out a window. My father, who was in town for a visit, went into Westley and Erik's bedroom to find the boys; he didn't see them behind the window curtain, where they were hiding. Taking a break from hide-and-seek, my father sat down in the living room to talk to me. Suddenly, we heard crying and screaming in the backyard.

We were dumbfounded on how the boys had gotten there, given that there wasn't a door in the back of the house—until we realized that their weight had pushed out the window screen, causing them to fall backwards out the window. Fortunately, we lived in a one-story house. Nonetheless, Erik had fractured his left arm and elbow, while Westley had fractured his left wrist. Their injuries made the boys the talk of the school. When I brought them to their classrooms after they had their casts put on, it was priceless to see the reactions and double takes of the other students. It was of course far less amusing to later see Westley's test scores. I hoped the cast was to blame.

Fifth Grade

As my boys entered fifth grade, I was already thinking ahead to another milestone: I couldn't believe that my boys would start middle school in one year. I was determined to make this fifth grade really count to get the boys on track.

School had only been in session for a week when I went to New York for my sister's wedding. I was gone five days. My husband brought the kids with him to pick me up at the airport. I hardly recognized Westley. He had severe facial tics, and his face was in spasm. I had never witnessed anything like it. Chris and I knew that it was probably stress; Westley had just started a new school year, and I had been away from him only once before, several years ago. Fortunately, the tics subsided over the next few days.

Westley's handwriting remained illegible most of the time. His fifth grade teacher was very patient with him. She said that when he slowed down and made an effort, he could produce excellent work. He continued to be a great writer with many creative ideas. But his teacher was still concerned about his organization skills and neatness, especially in math operations such as division and fractions.

Erik had many friends and loved school. In spite of his hyperactivity and distractibility, he was succeeding in the classroom. His teacher had a great sense of humor, which kept his interest. He continued to excel in history and did well in all other subjects. It seemed that my husband had been right about Ritalin. There was not enough of a problem to warrant it, though Erik's motor mouth was still very much present.

Westley was beginning to make new friends. But he still was overly eager to please his peers, which made him an easy target for some of the meaner kids. They would dare him to do silly things, and in an attempt to fit in, he would do them. When the recess bell rang, the children were to walk to get in line with their classmates. Kids would dare Westley to run and scream while going to the class line. And he'd do it, even as the other students laughed at him. On top of that, Erik would tell me that his brother frequently talked to himself at school, and some kids couldn't resist teasing him.

One boy named Wesley was a bit more mature than the rest. He would tell Westley that he had a choice, that he did not have to listen to those kids. He turned out to be Westley's best friend that year.

Westley still remained irritable at home, and we were constantly breaking up fights between him and Erik. Erik would tease Westley, and then Westley would physically attack him. Sometimes, if Erik just looked at him with an odd expression, Westley would fly off the handle. He never seemed happy. Going out to dinner or on vacations would often turn into a disaster. There was always a dark cloud around him. My husband and I were becoming very concerned because Westley was now physically strong and capable of causing serious injury to his brother. We hesitated to seek therapy—we didn't want to hear the Ritalin rap again.

A well-known homeopathic (natural medicine) practitioner in Santa Monica—Dr. Murray Clarke—was recommended to me. Many parents had turned to him while seeking alternative ways to address their children's ADHD diagnosis.

Dr. Clarke observed Westley and Erik and took a hair analysis to check for toxic elements and heavy metal poisoning. He ordered blood work to test for food allergies and examine their general blood chemistry. The results of the hair analysis showed a high level of lead, especially with Erik. Their general blood chemistry was within normal range. The food allergy test for Westley indicated a peanut allergy. Erik's test showed he had an allergy to peanuts, gluten, and garlic. Unfortunately, we couldn't continue to take the kids to the homoeopathic doctor—our insurance wouldn't cover it.

I showed their pediatrician the test results. He didn't give much weight to the hair analysis, but he did order a finger-prick blood test to check lead levels. Normal levels fall between one to nine micrograms per deciliter (mcg/dl). Westley's test showed four mcg/dl. Erik's test came back with an eight mcg/dl, a little on the high side but still in the normal range. The doctor wanted to recheck Erik's lead level in a few months.

I told my own doctor about the results, and he suggested that I give Erik 2,000 milligrams of Vitamin C a day to help remove the lead from his system (a process called detoxification). His lead level was checked two months later; it had dropped from eight mcg/dl to two mcg/dl.

Although the boys' lead levels fell within the normal range, there may be reason to doubt that "normal" and "healthy" are the same thing. An episode of PBS's acclaimed *Now* series, hosted by Bill Moyers, cited studies indicating that lead levels as low as three mcg/dl can impair a child's health. Another study, published in the *New England Journal of Medicine*, found that even lead levels below the federal and international guidelines of ten micrograms per deciliter produce a large drop in IQ— up to 7.4 points. Disturbingly, researchers estimate that one out of every ten U.S. children has levels of five mcg/dl or above.

Having addressed the boys' lead levels, I wanted to seek solutions to other problems, too. Because of his allergy, I tried to get Erik off wheat products; it was impossible. He complained it was bad enough that I'd taken dairy away from him. His health was good, and he had an excellent school attendance record, so I let it slide.

Meanwhile, Westley continued to exhibit facial tics, and I wanted to seek medical help for him. I took him to a neurologist. His symptoms were mild. She didn't observe any neurological problems and agreed the tics were stress related. I noticed that when he had problems with the kids at school, the severity of his facial tics would increase. He would do anything to make friends. He was easily led and quite naïve. Westley would get into more trouble than the kids who were daring him. He could not comprehend that the children were laughing at him and that they weren't really his friends. His behavior was becoming even more eccentric, and he didn't fit in with the other kids. When Westley did make a friend, the other kids would tease the student, and that would put an end to it. I couldn't even begin to imagine what it was going to be like in middle school.

Away from school, he would attack Erik over little things. Westley had a sweet side, but he often gave in to rage. He had absolutely no impulse control. Erik was beginning to fear him.

I had yet another reason to worry: Westley was shutting me out. He used to share his feelings with me. Now he would tell me that he was fine even though it was obvious he was not. I told him that I loved him unconditionally and that he could tell me anything. I was there to help. He needed an ally more than ever.

Westley was becoming more withdrawn and had a new obsession: *Dragon Ball Z*. He drew hundreds of sketches of the cartoon characters. The drawings were quite good, considering how terrible his handwriting was. He played with the *Dragon Ball Z* figures and chewed on the top of their heads. I took the figures away from him. He would throw a tantrum and promise not to chew on them, but without even realizing it himself, he would put toys right back in his mouth.

Both my husband and I were very baffled as to why Westley was so angry. We were aware that he might be jealous of his brother, but he had everything a child could need. We were a loving and supporting family. I was thinking it was possible that his irritability came from spending the first months of his life so ill. Being on a ventilator and being gavage-fed may have left some deep negative psychological impact on him. Perhaps there was something wrong with the wiring in his brain from being born so prematurely. We had no choice but to look into family counseling. Hoping that a psychotherapist would know how to reach him, we began family counseling at the Vista Del Mar Child and Family Services. The boys enjoyed the sessions. They both expressed their feelings well, but Westley continued to exhibit an angry attitude, while Erik was always fidgety.

Fifth grade flew by so fast. Having their elementary school right behind our house had been a great experience, and I was a bit overwhelmed by the thought of the boys going to middle school, where there were more than 1,800 students. Westley was still weak in areas of organization and neatness. I was also concerned for him socially. I know how awfully mean middle school kids can be. According to his teacher, he had made good academic progress, although his Stanford 9 scores did not reflect his teacher's findings. His spelling score remained very high, in the eighty-first percentile. The total reading score was very poor, in the twenty-fourth percentile; his math scores were in the twenty-first percentile, and his total language score had bottomed out in the ninth percentile.

The summer going into sixth grade was a busy one. We were moving again, and we continued family therapy. At the end of the family counseling session the psychotherapist asked me in private if I had ever heard of Asperger's syndrome. She described it as a high-functioning type of autism, suggested that Westley be evaluated for it, and recommended that I read *Asperger's Syndrome: A Guide for Parents and Professionals* by Tony Attwood (Jessica Kingsley Publishers, 1998). After reading the book, I thought there was a strong possibility that Westley did have it, even though he did not exhibit all the symptoms. He didn't lack empathy, which was one of the characteristics of Asperger's, but he was quite naïve and had little ability to form friendships. At times he exhibited repetitive speech and obsessed on his latest fixation. He was very clumsy and had odd postures, all symptoms of Asperger's. I took him to be evaluated by a licensed clinical psychologist. Her diagnostic impressions were as follows:

1. Asperger's syndrome
2. Expressive language disorder
3. Phonological disorder
4. Learning disorder, not otherwise specified

After receiving the report I spoke with the psychologist. She told me that while Westley exhibited Asperger-like symptoms, he had more of a social learning disability; unlike Asperger's sufferers, Westley did desire emotional connection. No matter what the official diagnosis was, I was very concerned that Westley was entering middle school with very little educational support. Being his mother, I could not help feeling a great deal of guilt. I blamed myself for letting him fall through the cracks. I would have to act quickly to get the services he needed.

Sixth Grade

Both Chris and I knew that Westley was going to need help and possibly be medicated for his anger. I had him assessed by a psychiatrist to consider a medicine trial. Her diagnosis included ADHD, Asperger's syndrome,

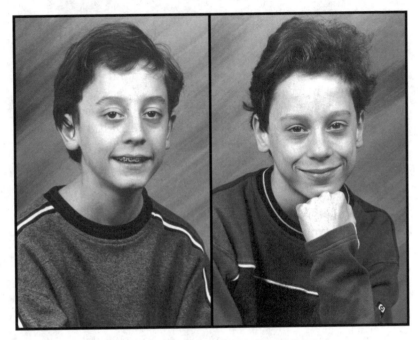

Erik and Westley in sixth grade.

and oppositional disorder. She was reluctant to prescribe Ritalin because of his facial tics, which were quite apparent in our sessions with her. After researching all the different medicines, we decided to try a drug called Risperdal (generically known as risperidone). It would address both his attention disorder and irritability, and it was not a stimulant.

As soon as school started, I requested an emergency Individualized Education Program meeting. The guidance counselor was helpful and set up an academic performance test. Westley's math scores were very weak, and he qualified for a math resource at school.

The Individualized Education Program meeting was held in November. It was decided that Westley would continue with adaptive P.E. and a weekly full-inclusion teacher would visit his classroom to assist his other teachers. His handwriting was so poor that we requested he receive an AlphaSmart keyboard to type all his work. The school said he no longer qualified for speech therapy, although he could not be understood a quarter of the time. The public school system could only do so much to address his needs.

Erik sailed beautifully into middle school. He was receiving all A's and B's except for math, where he was getting C's. His English teacher recommended him for the leadership program. He declined because he wanted to stay in chorus and he couldn't do both. He was making new friends. The only challenge that remained was getting him to do his homework.

Westley was receiving mostly C's in his classes. No one could read his handwriting, and the AlphaSmart keyboard never arrived as promised. Westley made a few friends in his adaptive P.E. class. He was a little upset and self-conscious because some children in the class were quite mentally handicapped. I told him that he could go into regular P.E. but also explained that it was very competitive. He decided to stay in adaptive P.E.

Some of the kids at school continued to make fun of Westley and dare him to do inappropriate things. One boy dared him to call his math teacher a bitch, and he did and received detention. He wrote his teacher a heartfelt apology letter, saying that he knew what he said was not true and he was very sorry. He blamed no one but himself.

The Risperdal did seem to take the edge off his anger. The boys would still fight, but not as often. The most negative side effect was that the medicine made Westley tired. He had a difficult time waking up in the morning even though he had enough sleep. We knew that the Risperdal was only going to be a temporary solution.

Still researching natural health and alternative medicine, I began to suspect that Westley might have candida albicans—an overgrowth of a common yeast in the intestines. Symptoms of yeast-connected problems are fatigue, irritability, short attention span, headaches, and respiratory problems, just to name a few. One of the causes of this condition is the overuse of antibiotics. His medical file showed he had experienced thirty-five rounds of antibiotics before he was six years old. He was still taking antibiotics frequently for his countless sinus infections.

My children's pediatrician was not knowledgeable about alternative medicine, so I asked my own doctor to order a candida test for Westley. The test results came back showing that his candida was abnormally high in all three categories he was tested for, including: IgG candida (blood long-term infection), IgM candida (acute candida infection), and IgA candida (infection in the gastro-intestinal tract and the bowels). My doctor prescribed nystatin, an anti-fungal medicine.

In addition to antibiotics, sugar can also cause an overgrowth of yeast in the intestines. I made an effort to feed my kids organic fruit after school instead of sweets. We would allow them to have soda when we went out to dinner, a once-a-week occurrence.

One of these restaurant excursions resulted in an eye-opening experience. Westley had spaghetti and a soft drink for dinner. He began to act silly and had his knife on his lap. I asked him to put the knife on his plate. He did, then smiled, and put his fork on his lap. I wasn't amused—and became even less so when he used my sleeve to wipe his face. I realized at this point that he was intoxicated on wheat and sugar. My husband had been in the restroom while this behavior was going on. Westley managed to pull himself together as his father dragged him out of the restaurant.

Often, the connection between the boys' behavior and what they ate was readily apparent. I avoided taking them to the supermarket, where they would beg me to buy junk food—exactly the type of food that could have the most nightmarish effect on their behavior. When they were eleven, Erik talked me into buying a multicolored fruit-flavor bar. At home, after eating only half their treats, both boys became hyperactive and out of control. I was confronted with two "Tasmanian Devils," and it was obvious to me that their behavior was connected to what they had just eaten. I threw the rest of the bars away after looking at the nutritional information on the box. The ingredients: water, sugar, corn syrup, high fructose corn syrup, natural and artificial flavoring, citric acid, guar gum, locust bean, Red No. 40, Blue No. 1, and Yellow Nos. 5 and 6. I have since learned that artificial food colors have been linked to allergies, asthma, and hyperactivity; they are also a possible carcinogenic.

Sixth grade was over, and Westley had straight C's, except for a D in math and an A in his keyboard class. The Stanford 9 results were encouraging. Westley's math score was in the fortieth percentile—quite an improvement from the year before, when his scores hit the twenty-first percentile. His reading score also increased, from the twenty-fourth percentile to the thirty-third. The greatest improvement was in his language skills, which had ranked in the ninth percentile in fifth grade—and which were now the fortieth percentile. He scored in the fifty-second percentile in language mechanics. I was relieved.

Erik's Stanford 9 results were all above average except for his spelling and math scores, which ranked in the twenty-second and thirty-eight percentile, respectively.

The psychotherapist recommended that I enroll Westley in a social skills group with psychologist Carol Hirschfield. She had developed the group for children who faced challenges like Westley's. The psychotherapist suggested it would help Westley improve his relations with his peers. I enrolled both of the boys. Erik loved it; Westley hated it. He would rather be home playing computer games or watching his favorite TV show, *Seventh Heaven*. I begged him to give the social skills group a chance, and after one month, if he was still unhappy, he could stop going.

We decided to take Westley off the Risperdal. He was just too tired every morning, even though he was on a very low dosage. He was still exhibiting facial tics. I was more than ever on my alternative medicine mission and knew there had to be something more natural that could help him without negative side effects.

Seventh Grade: Finding Answers

The boys continued with their weekly social skills group after school started. Westley would protest as we drove to the sessions, and he would argue with Erik on the way to the group and on the way home. I knew it was going to take a lot of persuading to make him keep going. So I decided that if the kids earned enough points, they would be able to pick out a toy at the end of the session. Unfortunately, Westley never earned enough points, which agitated him that much more. Even so, the group provided a safe environment for the kids to express themselves and discuss their everyday problems.

Erik's ongoing chattering remained one of his biggest challenges. He had a loud voice, and I could hear him talking while I sat in the waiting room. Once, I heard him complaining about me. He was angry at how fanatical I had become about his diet and vitamin supplements. He was sick of it and said it was not helping because he was still too skinny.

One afternoon I had Erik join me while I walked the dog. He spent the whole time telling me off. All his friends ate junk food and dairy products, he said, and they were healthy. He was embarrassed by how strict I was and was going to eat whatever he wanted from now on, including hotdogs (which are loaded with nitrates which can cause behavior problems and known to be carcinogenic). Erik ended the conversation by telling me that other than the "diet stuff," he still liked me. He was making me laugh and cry at the same time.

Westley was falling flat on his face in seventh grade. His handwriting looked like scribbling. He would start writing in the middle of the page, and the words would run together. It was impossible to read what he wrote. The full-inclusion teacher repeatedly told me she was working to get him an AlphaSmart keyboard. Westley began to give up. He would rather not try at all than to try and fail. His teacher said he was missing assignments and that the work he turned in wasn't acceptable.

There was always a lot of pressure connected with getting the boys ready for school. Erik would sneak away from his breakfast to watch cartoons. He would wait to the very last second to get dressed. One morning both children were running very late, and I heard a commotion going on upstairs. The boys were fighting, and I broke them up and hurried them out the front door so they wouldn't miss their ride to school. I picked them up after school, and Erik came out first. There were severe red scratches all across his face. "What did you tell your friends about your face?" I asked him. He'd told them he had fallen and scratched himself. Then Westley came out, looking no better than his brother. "What did you tell *your* friends?" I asked. His answer had been more straightforward: he'd told them that he got into a cat fight with his brother.

The boys were not getting along at all. And Erik was becoming more aggressive out of self-defense. I was at a loss and didn't know what to do next. I hoped that the social skills group would be able to help them work it out.

Erik was becoming more hyperactive. He would walk across the back of the couch or climb all over it as he watched television. The cushions would be thrown all over the room. At times he was not as hyper. I realized that when he was on antibiotics—particularly Zithromax (azithromycin)—his hyperactivity increased.

Westley's test scores were still very poor, mostly because of his handwriting. His science teacher gave him a zero on a test and, next to the grade, wrote, "I can't read this paper." He had been promised an AlphaSmart keyboard one year before. It finally arrived. It was defective, and it could not print out his work. It was November, and nothing was going right for him. He received an F on a history test. His teacher gave him a chance to retake the exam, but he didn't bother to study for it. He didn't seem to care anymore. His backpack was always filled with crinkled paper, bulging out of his folders. The only good news was that Westley wasn't getting as many respiratory infections as before. I thought that possibly the nystatin treatment for his candida was improving his health.

Other than the first several months after my children's birth, I was experiencing the darkest moments of my motherhood. I was confused and clueless as to what to do next to help Westley. I felt it was a hopeless situation. I had tried everything and at this point had to let go and put it into God's hands. After my kids left for school I sat down and prayed, fervently. My prayer was soon to be answered in a big way.

Feeling fatigued, anxious, and depressed, I went to see Dr. David Allen, MD, for an acupuncture treatment. He was already well aware of the situation with my children, and I told him how Westley's constant irritability and violent temper seemed to be getting worse. In response, Dr. Allen suggested that Westley undergo a Quantitative Electroencephalography (QEEG) "brain mapping" procedure to determine whether seizures were behind his behavior. We scheduled an appointment.

In the meantime, Westley's psychologist called me and told me that there was no way that the Los Angeles Unified School District could meet all of his needs. She told me about a non public private school called Village Glen. They had recently opened a campus not too far from our neighborhood. The school served children with social and communication disabilities, including high-functioning autism and Asperger's. Social skills and expressive language were emphasized in every class. I visited the campus the following week. I was impressed with the program as well as the staff. The school's capacity was 200 students. At the time there were only seventy-one students enrolled.

I contacted the Regional Center to have Westley evaluated one more time for Asperger's and for educational support. The same doctor did the evaluation, and said that Westley did not have Asperger's. Her diagnostic impressions:

1. Highly scattered cognitive abilities
2. Unclear articulation to the degree he is quite difficult to understand at least twenty-five percent of the time
3. Poor perception of body and space
4. History of facial tics; some periods of shuddering were observed
5. Impulsivity; social immaturity

At the follow-up with the doctor, she asked me whether anyone ever diagnosed Westley as having cerebral palsy. She said it could be connected to the neonatal risk factors, which probably contributed to articulation difficulties, gross motor awkwardness, and fine motor challenges. I told her that a pediatrician had ruled out cerebral palsy when he was two and a half years old because he had been walking in an age-appropriate manner. She then wondered whether his disabilities might have come from organic impairment, a result of the premature birth. Because Westley was very engaging during the assessment, she said the diagnosis of Asperger's was no longer appropriate. Regardless, we all believed that he would benefit from a school such as Village Glen to meet his needs with his expressive language delays and social learning disability.

Westley's psychologist attended the Individualized Education Program meeting to support us in getting the approval we needed from the school administration to let Westley go to Village Glen. All of his academic teachers reported that he had a great deal of difficulty paying attention and staying on task. He would become confused and forget what he was supposed to do on his assignments. He often would not be able to find his work in his messy backpack. He constantly needed one-on-one assistance from the teachers. He had a great deal of difficulty with visual-motor integration and auditory processing, which affected his ability to write notes, copy information, and express his thoughts in writing.

The occupational assessment reported that Westley's hand manipulation skills were in decline, as was his visual-motor control when performing handwriting activities; he could not read his own handwriting. He had trouble focusing on important points and tended to get hung up on irrelevant details. All the teachers were going out of their way to accommodate him in the class by photocopying other students' notes and giving him more time to complete the assignments. According to all his teachers, his main problem was missing work.

We also feared for Westley's safety. He had many challenges with impulse control. And the middle school kids were always trying to make him say and do mean things to the other students. If a child told him to kick someone, he would. He had difficulty in understanding social nuances. He just wanted to make friends to be accepted by his peers. For safety's sake we had to get him out of public middle school.

All the school staff members unanimously agreed that Los Angeles

Unified School District should let Westley attend a non-public school and that LAUSD should pay for it. We were very relieved; unfortunately, Westley was not crazy about the idea of leaving his few friends.

With all the problems in his current school, he still resisted going to Village Glen. There were two more weeks of class before winter break. He wanted to go back to his public school after winter break for three more weeks and finish out the semester. We allowed him to do so, and I assured him that if he was unhappy with Village Glen, he could always return to a public school.

Some of my siblings and good friends were concerned for Westley's lack of progress. They said I had waited long enough, and out of concern for him, they advised me to try a trial run of Ritalin. I thanked everyone for their concern and told them about the imminent QEEG brain map, which, we hoped, would offer some answers.

The day of Westley's appointment arrived. To begin the procedure, a technician pasted sensors on Westley's head that would record his brainwaves as he performed math problems, reading and other tasks. The machine also recorded his brainwaves as he shut his eyes and relaxed. One and a half hours later, the procedure was complete.

My husband and I went to Dr. Allen's office to get the test results. The QEEG report showed abnormal activity in Westley's brain. Frankly, we weren't surprised. His brain had a marked excess of episodic anterior high-voltage fast activity, as well as episodes of frontal dominant slow (theta) activity. In lay terms, parts of his brain were moving too slowly, while other parts were moving too fast. The doctor described it as playing a football game with all of the players running at different speeds. His brain was missing the relaxation type of rhythm, which created seizure-like activity in his brain. This discovery would explain why Westley was irritable so much of the time. He had a hyper-reactive brain with little threshold. According to our doctor, if we had put him on Ritalin or any other stimulant, it would have most likely made him worse or even had caused him to have a convulsion, one of the many side effects of the drug.

My husband's hunches were correct all along about not medicating Westley. Usually the anti-seizure medicine Depakote (generically known as divalproex sodium) would be recommended for Westley's type of brain activity. Depakote has many side effects, and our doctor said Westley

0011 Amino Acid Analysis - 20 Plasma	Results	Reference Limits (For adults 13 and over)	Low Limit	High Limit
Essential Amino Acids				
Arginine	90	70 - 160	70	160
Histidine	71	65 - 150	65	150
Isoleucine	51	50 - 160	50	160
Leucine	102 L	105 - 250	105	250
Lysine	138 L	140 - 250	140	250
Methionine	24	20 - 60	20	60
Phenylalanine	46	45 - 140	45	140
Threonine	109	85 - 250	85	250
Tryptophan	55	45 - 120	45	120
Valine	174 L	180 - 480	180	480
Essential Amino Acid Derivatives				umol/L
Neuroendocrine Metabolism			Low Limit	High Limit
Glycine	209	200 - 450	200	450
Serine	77 L	80 - 200	80	200
Taurine	50	50 - 250	50	250
Tyrosine	61	50 - 120	50	120
Ammonia/Energy Metabolism			Low Limit	High Limit
Asparagine	37	35 - 100	35	100
Aspartic Acid	9	6 - 30	6	30
Citrulline	38	15 - 70	15	70
Glutamic Acid	53	45 - 200	45	200
Glutamine	572	500 - 1,050	500	1050
Ornithine	82	35 - 100	35	100

Methodology: ION Exchange HPLC

Westley's amino acid profile.

should first undergo an amino acid panel test. Low amino acid levels could be contributing to his abnormal brain activity.

Chris took Westley in for the test the day after Christmas. In Westley's usual manner he created quite a scene at the doctor's office, throwing a tantrum as the nurse drew his blood.

Three agonizing weeks later, we received the test results. The test measures levels of twenty amino acids. Westley had four in the low range and sixteen in the medium-low range—a significant amino acid deficiency.

0011 Amino Acid Analysis - 20 Plasma			Methodology: ION Exchange HPLC
	Results	Reference Limits (For adults 13 and over)	

Essential Amino Acids

	Results	Reference Limits	Low Limit	High Limit
Arginine	84	70 - 160	70	160
Histidine	68	65 - 150	65	150
Isoleucine	49 L	50 - 160	50	160
Leucine	102 L	105 - 250	105	250
Lysine	133 L	140 - 250	140	250
Methionine	23	20 - 60	20	60
Phenylalanine	45	45 - 140	45	140
Threonine	84 L	85 - 250	85	250
Tryptophan	45	45 - 120	45	120
Valine	190	180 - 480	180	480

Essential Amino Acid Derivatives   umol/L

Neuroendocrine Metabolism

	Results	Reference Limits	Low Limit	High Limit
Glycine	228	200 - 450	200	450
Serine	97	80 - 200	80	200
Taurine	31 L	50 - 250	50	250
Tyrosine	61	50 - 120	50	120

Ammonia/Energy Metabolism

	Results	Reference Limits	Low Limit	High Limit
Asparagine	36	35 - 100	35	100
Aspartic Acid	7	6 - 30	6	30
Citrulline	22	15 - 70	15	70
Glutamic Acid	51	45 - 200	45	200
Glutamine	491 L	500 - 1,050	500	1050
Ornithine	54	35 - 100	35	100

Erik's amino acid profile.

Either Westley was not getting enough protein in his diet or he had poor digestive absorption. Dr. Allen prescribed four free-form amino acid capsules, to be taken on an empty stomach two times a day. He also prescribed additional amino acid supplements, including one taurine tablet, one GABA (gamma-aminobutyric acid) tablet, and two inositol tablets, to be taken with breakfast and dinner. Vitamin B6 was prescribed to help with the metabolism of the amino acids, and Dr. Allen suggested a multivitamin and cod liver oil (an essential fatty acid source) to help support the neuron connections in Westley's brain. The doctor said that we should start seeing an improvement within a few weeks.

I went home and read everything I could find in my nutrition books about amino acids. Westley was low in the amino acid lysine; low lysine levels could cause low energy, inability to concentrate, and irritability. Westley's taurine levels were also extremely low, a deficiency that could lead to tics, epilepsy, anxiety, hyperactivity, and poor brain function. Some of Westley's most significant challenges were symptoms of low amino acid levels.

Even so, I did not have any great expectations for a positive outcome. The other measures we had tried had helped somewhat—we'd removed dairy from his diet, addressed his candida with nystatin, and turned to Risperdal for his attention disorder and anger. Unfortunately, nothing to this point had made a big difference in his violent behavior, poor impulse control, impaired attention, or facial tics.

Yet after Westley's first week of taking the amino acid supplements, I noticed that there had been no bickering between the kids. This change was a miracle in itself. Moreover, Westley was going out of his way to talk to me after years of being distant and cranky. His psychologist commented on how much more Westley was participating in the social-skills group. The cloud was lifting from him. I was no longer observing facial tics or twitches. I knew that the amino acids were working.

Westley attended his new school in the beginning of February. The bus picked him up and dropped him off at our home. On the first day of school he was nervous. But he handled the transition very well. His class had nine students, one teacher, and an aide. The students welcomed him, and he made new friends in no time. He was where he was supposed to be.

After three weeks at his new school, he came home one afternoon, and when I opened the door, there stood Westley with a happy grin from ear to ear. He could not stop smiling. His voice brimming with emotion, he announced, "I love life!"

The amino acids were the missing link. He continued to improve in his school performance. His grades went from C's and D's to A's and B's. He was doing his homework independently. One Sunday, when he went up to his room for a couple of hours, I assumed he was playing computer games. Instead, he was typing his book report on his computer and printing it out without anyone's assistance. He received an A- on his report.

We were very proud of him.

Because an apple does not fall far from the tree, I thought it would be a good idea to have my and Erik's amino acid levels checked. I was shocked when the results came back. Our amino acid levels were lower than Westley's! I was not as surprised about Erik, because he is the pickier eater of the two. He had never cared for protein foods, such as poultry, fish, beef, beans, and nuts. Erik was at the bottom of the low on trypto-phan. Tryptophan is a precursor to serotonin and helps control hyperac-tivity in children. Erik had always been the more hyper one. He began taking a tryptophan supplement before bed and, after a week, calmed down substantially.

My own test results were alarming. Out of the twenty amino acids tested, thirteen were low. The remaining seven were in the medium-low range. I had a low-protein diet. With my stressful life the little protein that I was consuming would be immediately zapped up. I ordered a cus-tom-made amino acid compound. Dr. Allen also prescribed tyrosine, phenylalanine and glutamine. Within one week I felt an increase of en-ergy and I was more alert. Life didn't seem like such a burden anymore. I was experiencing firsthand Westley's happy mood. I actually felt giddy. I had no idea how depressed I had been all that time. I had been so overly consumed with my kids' issues that I had no energy or time to take care of myself.

The Boys Today

As I write this chapter the boys are at the end of eighth grade. They've taken amino acid supplements for more than one and a half years. West-ley continues to receive A's and B's on his report cards. At his school, he was awarded Most Improved Student of the year in behavior and social skills. He has not in a year and a half scratched, hit, kicked, or bitten his brother, though Erik continues to tease him relentlessly. The teasing up-sets Westley, but he expresses himself verbally instead of giving in to his impulses and becoming violent.

The good news doesn't stop there. I have not observed one facial tic or any twitches in Westley in the past one and a half years. He had symp-toms of an attention deficit, but it wasn't from a Ritalin deficiency—it stemmed from low neurotransmitter activity, caused by low amino acid levels.

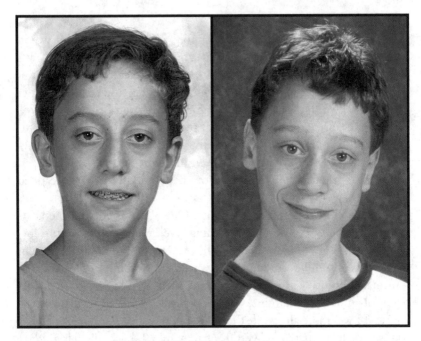

Erik and Westley in eighth grade.

In addition to taking supplements, my children continue to eat healthfully, avoiding foods that exacerbated their worst behaviors. It was no easy task to make dietary changes with my children. They were stubborn and picky eaters. I took them to natural food markets and allowed them to select some of the food items. Most delicatessens allow free samples for tasting. I was ultimately successful in changing the way my children eat because I made them a part of the process.

Looking Back
I initially thought all of my children's health issues and developmental delays were a result of their premature birth. Although premature infants are at risk for development delays, I now believe there were other contributing factors—such as vaccines.

And why? The measles-mumps-rubella vaccine is highly immunogenic, meaning it stimulates the immune system. Many children with ADHD, learning disabilities, and developmental delays also have autoimmune dysfunction, with several allergies to foods, drugs, and environmental toxins. One of the first things I learned in the NICU is that premature girls out survive premature boys—girls tend to have a stronger immune system. Might this be one reason why boys are diagnosed with autism and ADHD three to four times more than girls?

Numerous newspaper and magazine articles have questioned whether mercury in the environment and childhood vaccines (all contained mercury prior to 1999, and some still do) could be connected to autism and attention disorders. Aluminum is also used in some vaccines. Mercury and aluminum toxicity has been linked to arthritis, asthma, allergies, Alzheimer's, diabetes, multiple sclerosis, fibromyalgia, lupus, chronic fatigue syndrome, depression, bipolar disorder, schizophrenia, and learning disabilities.

In their excellent book *A Shot in the Dark* (Avery Publishing, 1991), authors Harris L. Coulter and Barbara Loe Fisher list several circumstances indicating when a vaccine should be withheld:

- A history of seizures or other neurological diseases in the child or other member of the immediate family
- A history of allergy to components used in the vaccines, such as eggs, gelatin, casein, or thimersal (which contains mercury)
- Premature or low birth weight
- A chronic or recent illness
- A parent or sibling with a vaccine reaction
- A prior severe reaction to a vaccination

If I had known then what I know now, I would not have had my sons vaccinated: they had been born prematurely, their birth weights were low, and Westley had hyaline membrane disease. They both have asthma, symptoms of ADHD, and allergies to many foods, medicines, and environmental toxins. I can't help but wonder whether vaccinating my children contributed to many of these problems. Heavy-metal tests in both of my children indicated aluminum and mercury were present, though not in the very elevated range. Regardless, there is no "safe" level for any heavy metal. Fortunately, supplementing Erik and Westley's diet with amino acids and Vitamin C helped lower their levels of toxic heavy metals.

When I sought help for my kids' issues, Ritalin was always cast as the solution—the only solution. The doctors would evaluate Erik and Westley for twenty minutes and tell us that they needed to go on Ritalin. Not one of the psychiatrists, psychologists, or medical doctors ever addressed their diets or other possible causes. When I would ask them whether the boys' diet could be causing their symptoms, the reply would be that diet had nothing to do with it and the cause was probably a chemical imbalance in the brain.

Westley's symptoms worsened as he got older. It was frightening to imagine where he could have wound up in life—he had been failing in school and was being easily led by the wrong kids. His violent temper and poor impulse control had been a great challenge for him. His facial tics were always present. I feared for him. What would have happened had he not undergone a QEEG or an amino acid test? Would he have run into trouble with the law? Would he have ultimately ended up in jail? I don't know, and I'm still frustrated: overall (excepting the intensive neonatal care) that the conventional medical establishment failed my children—and me.

Chapter 2
From Sickness to Health:
My Own Journey

As I noted earlier, the apple doesn't fall far from the tree: like my children, I have had the symptoms of an attention disorder my whole life. But I never had a label for my problems—until I learned about my kids' disorder.

Much of my life was spent struggling against attention problems—in addition to other health challenges, including frequent infections. In trying to get healthy, I saw doctor after doctor and ingested a pharmacological cornucopia of medicines—without luck.

It was only after turning to natural medicine solutions and natural living that I began to transform my health. Today, after many years of suffering, I am finally strong, healthy, and happy.

A Lifetime of Illness

I remember how hard it was to pay attention in school. My greatest fear was that I wouldn't pass to the next grade level. Teachers frequently caught me daydreaming. In elementary school, although I did well on spelling tests and loved drawing, I was a slow reader, and math was challenging. I was also uncoordinated; in P.E., I was often the last kid picked to play on a team. I had a speech impediment, which the other kids teased me about, I was immature for my age, and my friendships never

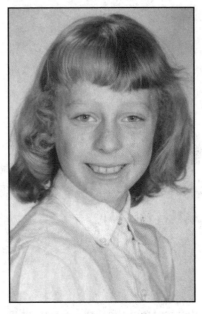

Fourth grade

lasted long. I became a loner and suffered from low self-esteem.

To make matters worse, I was in a prestigious public school system in Ridgewood, New Jersey. Passing eighth grade became an uphill battle. Then, new problems emerged, compounding my academic difficulties: I started to experience regular respiratory infections, and teachers often told me that I looked tired.

By ninth grade, my family had moved to a new school district, and I was bringing my grades up (except in algebra, which I never passed). But my health problems persisted. My senior year, I began feeling weak and had low energy. My doctor ordered a general blood chemical panel. The test results indicated low thyroidal activity. Though a CAT scan was ordered, I never saw the results—the hospital lost my records, and I moved away to college without seeking additional medical attention for my thyroid.

In my early twenties, I was being treated for bronchitis when my doctor noticed a large goiter in my neck. A CAT scan indicated that I had hypothyroidism—an underactive thyroid. I was prescribed Synthroid (levothyroxine sodium), which I took until I was thirty years old. A doctor took me off the medicine to retest my thyroid; the test results showed it to be functioning within normal ranges.

Other than having an occasional respiratory infection and still experiencing the challenges of an undiagnosed attention disorder, my health was stable for several years—until my children began preschool. My immune system took hit after hit. I was catching all of their infections; I had frequent ear infections and chronic bronchitis. The medicines I was prescribed created new problems. Every time I took penicillin, bumps appeared on my fingers. My doctor switched me to the combination antibiotic Bactrim (sulfamethoxazole and trimethoprim). It didn't take much time for hives to appear on my arms. I was prescribed other antibiotics but had to go off them after a few days because of negative side effects.

Meanwhile, as doctors were recommending Ritalin for my children, I began wondering about my own attention disorder. Although my husband was opposed to Ritalin for Erik and Westley, I wanted to try it myself to see if it would alleviate my own behavioral challenges. After a psychiatric examination, I was prescribed Ritalin. But it was difficult to determine whether it was helping—I was chronically sick with ear infections, bronchitis, and chronic fatigue.

That's when the behavior specialist I was seeing for Westley and Erik suggested that I try an antidepressant. She said it would help take the edge off the stress of raising ADHD-diagnosed twins. I stopped Ritalin and was prescribed Zoloft. Within three days of taking the drug, my sex drive disappeared. My emotions felt as though they were trapped in a cave inside my brain. I was numb. The medicine actually made me depressed. I stopped Zoloft after a month. Soon afterward, I was diagnosed with Hashimoto's thyroiditis, an underactive thyroid disorder. I began taking Synthroid again.

At the same time, my ear infections were so persistent that I was experiencing vertigo. (One night, I became so dizzy that I couldn't walk two feet without losing my balance. I was worried: I had completed a course of antibiotics—and I still felt sick.) I often heard a loud ringing in my years, and my brain felt fuzzy. I also suffered numerous respiratory infections as well as environmental allergies and chronic headaches. I frequently complained to my husband that my brain felt toxic. I never felt well.

My doctor prescribed me Cipro (ciprofloxacin), yet another antibiotic. Days after I began taking it, my husband noticed a white patch on my cheek. I didn't give it much thought because I am so pale to begin with. A few months later, I began another round of Cipro. Within two days, I lost 30 percent of my pigmentation. White blotches covered my body. My dermatologist diagnosed me with vitiligo, an autoimmune disease that affects 1 to 2 percent of the population.

At this point, I had had enough of doctors who were bound to the Western tradition of medicine. I was determined to find a medical doctor who practiced alternative medicine.

The Turning Point

My first encounter with non-Western medical care was with the Traditional Chinese Medical (TCM) doctor, who succeeded in treating our ear infections by warning us to not consume dairy products.

At about that time, I had read *The Yeast Syndrome,* a book by John Parks Trowbridge and Morton Walker, DPM. It struck a chord. Candida, the book reported, could exhaust the endocrine system and lead to many conditions, including two I'd been diagnosed with: hypothyroidism and vitiligo. Frequent use of antibiotics could cause candida, as could a diet like mine—one high in sugar.

It was difficult to find a physician who believed that candida even existed, let alone one who knew how to treat it. I was finally referred to Dr. David Allen, MD, who practices both conventional and alternative medicine. In my first visit to his office, he explained that a pregnancy can deplete a woman's body of nutrients and send her immune system on a downward spiral. It made sense to me, especially as a mother of twins whose behavior and health issues had put a lot of stress on my immune system.

I underwent several tests, including one for candida, which indicated that my candida levels were indeed high. Dr. Allen prescribed nystatin, an antifungal medicine. I went on the candida diet, which is not an easy task—but I wanted to get well. To get rid of candida, many foods must be eliminated from the diet, such as sugar, wheat, rye, dairy, mushrooms, alcohol, all junk food, refined food, artificial sweeteners and fermented foods like vinegar and soy sauce.

But my candida wouldn't budge. If anything, it was getting worse. I took myself off nystatin after one year. But I didn't give up.

The Next Steps

Plagued with allergies, vitiligo, and Hashimoto's thyroiditis, I attended a medical lecture featuring a panel of doctors, one of whom spoke about autoimmune diseases—and offered a warning that would change my life: "If you are in your thirties and forties and have been suffering from autoimmune diseases," he said, "it may be connected to the amalgam fillings in your mouth."

Amalgam fillings. One of my earliest memories involved going to the dentist—I had plenty of cavities. They were filled with amalgam: silvery metal containing mercury. By adulthood, I had fifteen mercury amalgam fillings in my mouth.

I never thought much about my metal filings until I was in my early twenties—when I began hearing a strange buzzing noise in my head as I fell asleep. It was scary, but I could stop the buzzing if I forced myself to wake up. As soon as I started to go back to sleep, the buzzing would return. I would try to wake back up, but I'd be too exhausted, almost as though I were paralyzed. I would awaken the next morning feeling okay but baffled by what had occurred.

One afternoon as I lay down to nap, I again heard buzzing—but, I decided not to fight the noise. To my surprise, *I tuned into a radio station.* The sound was clear and loud.

Befuddled, I told a friend about the experience. He speculated that the silver in my fillings could act as an antenna—I could have picked up radio waves. I talked to my dentist, who confirmed that there were documented cases of amalgam fillings tuning into radio frequencies. The mystery was solved, and, coincidentally, the buzzing sound never returned.

After hearing the doctor's warning against amalgam, it was clear that it was time to start thinking about my fillings again. They'd been the culprit behind the mysterious buzzing in my head when I was in my twenties—could they also be behind the mystery of my impaired immune system? I had already read in alternative medicine books that mercury contributes to candida. I knew I had to take action and figure out whether mercury was damaging my health.

Soon after the lecture, I had my body tested for heavy metals with the urine toxic element DMPS (dimethyl mercapto propionic acid) test. The results showed my mercury levels were in a highly elevated range. I never ate fish, so I knew my amalgam fillings were the source of the mercury poisoning in my body.

Over the next several months, I had all my fillings removed and replaced with composite material. I never again experienced another toxic headache. I later had several DMPS IVs (chelation therapy treatments) to help my body detox from mercury.

Afterward, I began having fewer respiratory infections, and my environmental allergies no long bothered me. My energy increased. I then began to take an antifungal medicine, Diflucan (fluconazole). Finally, after eight years of vitiligo, a significant amount of my skin's pigmentation returned.

About that time, as I discussed earlier, Dr. Allen was testing Westley for amino acid deficiencies—a lack of amino acids in the diet, or difficulty digesting amino acids, could precipitate exactly the sort of attention and behavioral problems Westley had experienced for years. The test results showed that Westley's amino acid levels were indeed low. I wondered about Erik's—and my own. Sure enough, tests showed that our amino acid levels were low, too.

A compound pharmacy created a custom amino acid compound to address my exact deficiency. To help in metabolizing these amino acids, I took Vitamin B6. As with Erik and Westley, the results were amazing. *Supplementing my diet with amino acids elevated my energy and general health to a level that I never before experienced.* I found it much easier to focus and was able to better handle everyday stress.

Please see the Resources Chapter for supplement information and laboratories that conduct tests for amino acids, heavy metals, pesticides, other toxins, and candida.

Why Me?

As I think back to childhood, I have many revelations as to what caused my persistent illnesses and attention disorder. The amalgam fillings constituted one factor. I also believe my poor diet, which once included far too much sugar, further hampered my health.

I was born with an insane addiction to sugar. My mother kept few sweets in the house; unfortunately, that did not stop me form making sugar the staple of my diet. I recall walking one mile to the corner store, when I was as young as seven years old, because a quarter would buy me five candy bars. I made sure that I ate them all before I got home so my mother would not find out about my sweet secret. Since then, I've learned a lot about sugar—particularly how it can encourage candida growth and how it negatively affects mood, attention, and behavior.

Beyond the fillings and the sugar, I've concluded that the exposure to pesticides during my childhood also impaired my health. In the 1950's and 1960's, when I was growing up, trucks drove down our streets and sprayed insecticides on the trees to kill mosquitoes. I spent a lot of time as a young girl outside, climbing trees and exploring nature. I remember seeing pesticide residue dripping from the trees I climbed.

In exploring natural health issues, I have learned that some of the common symptoms of pesticide poisoning include an inability to think, poor concentration, hyperactivity, poor coordination, weakness, nervousness, breathing problems, muscle pains, and twitching—the symptoms we associate with a number of neurological challenges, including ADHD. Fortunately, in the 1960's, people became alarmed over the amount of insecticides being used and their effect on animals and people—thanks in large part to Rachel Carson's book, *Silent Spring* (Houghten Mifflin Company 1962). The U.S. government began to gradually phase out all uses of DDT in 1972. In 1975, most uses of chlordane were banned.

Staying Healthy

To get and stay well I had to become proactive in educating myself. I read books on alternative medicine, attended lectures, and listened carefully to alternative medicine practitioners—all of which has led me to adopt the natural living lifestyle.

To help detox from toxins I use chlorella algae, which has been proven to bind with and remove toxic metals and pesticides from the body. I also use cilantro for detoxification purposes. To support my brain, adrenals, and thyroid, I take essential fatty acids such as flaxseed oil and evening primrose. I no longer take Synthroid because it is synthetic and often ineffective. Instead, I use a raw thyroid glandular. To prevent recurring candida, I take acidophilus to balance my intestinal flora and natural antifungal supplements such as olive leaf extract.

I buy organic produce. I eat raw food as much as possible. For breakfast, I mix two tablespoons of Dr. Schulze's Superfood in a glass of vegetable juice. Dr. Schulze's Superfood is 100 percent organic with whole food and herbal vitamins and minerals (see www.herbdoc.com). The ingredients are spirulina, blue-green algae, chlorella, alfalfa, barley, wheatgrass, purple dulse seaweed, beetroot, spinach leaf, rosehips, orange peel, lemon peel, and non-active *Saccharomyces cervisiae* nutritional yeast. Because the Superfood is made of numerous single-celled micro-plants, the body is able to assimilate it in minutes, right into the blood. I have not had one infection since supplementing my diet with Superfood.

The lesson I learned through my journey to get well is that *there was no magic pill to cure me.* I had to address many conditions to bring my body to a healthy state. Detoxing from mercury and other toxins, along

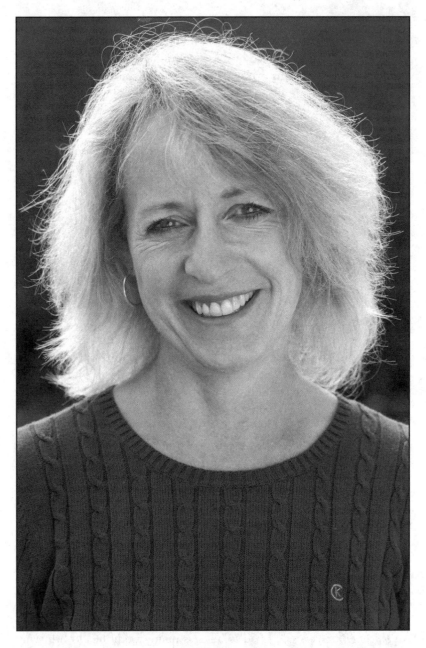

"You CAN have victory over ADHD—just like we did!"

with major diet changes, supplements (particularly amino acid supplements), and eating real, *alive* food—not processed *dead* food—made the difference.

I hope you'll use this book to find what will make the difference for you.

The second part of this book provides an overview of the possible causes of attention disorders, autism, and other neurological disorders. Alternative solutions for healing are covered, as well as resources for supplements and laboratories that conduct tests for amino acids, heavy metals, pesticides, other toxins, and candida. May you be inspired to adopt these suggestions for the total healing of yourself, your children and your family—you now know it's worth the effort.

Chapter 3
The Problems With Conventional Medicine

For treatment of chronic conditions, the allopathic (meaning, conventional) medical approach taught at most medical schools—and practiced by the majority of medical doctors—relies on identifying diseases or symptoms, then prescribing drugs to manage or combat those conditions. It is a belief system that considers the disease or symptom to be the *actual problem*, as opposed to addressing the *underlying causes* that produced the disease or symptom in the first place.

There exists a wide variety of tests, procedures, and equipment specially designed to identify diseases and symptoms. While these tools *could* be used in discerning the underlying causes of chronic illness, they rarely are. Instead, once a diagnosis is determined, test results are frequently plunked into the patient's file as conclusive evidence of his or her condition. The allopathic medical practitioner then attempts to manage that condition, usually with drugs. This chapter enumerates the reasons why the conventional medical approach ultimately cheats people who are seeking a health solution—be it for an ordinary cold or a neurological problem such as ADD/ADHD.

Treating Symptoms Instead of Causes

Consider ear infections, a common affliction in American children (ninety-five percent of children before the age of five have had an ear infection). The allopathic model recommends treatment with antibiotics. That's treating the symptom. The infection may go away, but the underlying cause of the infection could still exist—and even worsen with continued reliance on antibiotics. Antibiotic use not only destroys offending bacteria in the ear, but also kills immune-building bacteria in the gut, creating a spiraling effect of ear infections and antibiotic treatment.

This can lead to even more ear infections and severely compromise the inner ear—which affects more than the ability to hear. The inner ear houses the vestibular system, which provides us with the ability to process information about movement, gravity, balance, and space—in short, it monitors everything we *do*. It is foundational to many other neurodevelopmental systems and therefore enables us to multi-track. A weakness in vestibular/inner ear functioning can cause pervasive problems, including issues and challenges seen in adults and children diagnosed with ADD/ADHD.[1]

With overall health in mind, the natural medical practitioner will look beyond symptoms—and question why the immune system has weakened to such a degree that an ear infection could occur. The underlying cause may be an allergy, such as to dairy; poor nutrition; excessive sugar consumption; fluoride poisoning (a chemical that in sufficient concentration damages the immune system and interferes with enzyme production); or stress (in utero, during birth, and/or after birth).[2] Other factors influencing ear infections include structural irregularities in the ear, as well as irregularities with the endolymphatic sac and its articulation with the dura mater (the outer meningeal lining of the brain).

Whatever the cause, the natural doctor seeks to identify it and address it—strengthening the immune system as she treats the symptoms of the infection. Treatment of the ear infection itself may include the use of homeopathy and/or nontoxic herbal formulas, such as garlic and mullein, to subdue harmful bacteria. This natural medicine stops the current ear infection and improves the immune system to treat an underlying cause—making future ear infections very unlikely.

Reliance on Drug Therapies

Drugs—when used for chronic conditions (as opposed to acute trauma conditions)—are almost always designed to control or manage certain bodily systems for the long term. They have serious side effects if they are toxic to the body. For example, Ritalin and other stimulant medications may *artificially* speed up neurological processing so that a child or adult can function more "normally." The downfall is that the underlying causes of slow or disordered neurological functioning are never addressed. In addition, the child may suffer horrible side effects—which are in fact evidence of drug poisoning.

In certain situations, drugs may be required for short-term use. But long-term use can produce even more problems from side effects. Meanwhile, underlying conditions go unnoticed and untreated, and overall functioning may deteriorate further. From an allopathic perspective, this deterioration would require even more drug intervention, leading to an escalating spiral of medication and adverse reactions to the medications. Bottom line: when drugs are used to treat symptoms and no further action is taken to understand and treat the underlying cause, the problem, or problems, may worsen.

Overuse of Antibiotics

Antibiotics are prescribed to treat bacterial infections (and at times even viral infections, though they don't work against viruses). While antibiotics may occasionally be useful for life-threatening illnesses, their continual use will make some antibiotics ineffective, and more importantly, they can seriously compromise the body's immune system by destroying friendly bacteria in the gut. In fact, as is often seen with children with ear infections, antibiotics may kill the offending bacteria in the ear, but will also kill the friendly bacteria required to build the immune system. The destruction of friendly bacteria can lead to an overgrowth of unfriendly bacteria, such as candida, which is known to cause a plethora of other health problems (e.g., leaky gut syndrome, food intolerances, and overall nutritional deficits).

From a natural medicine perspective, bacteria don't "cause" an ear infection; the "cause" is frequently a weakened immune system that can't prevent the bacteria from multiplying, since bacteria are around us all the time. When antibiotics are prescribed for each recurring ear infection, the immune system is compromised a little more, requiring even more use of antibiotics for each new infection. This vicious ear infection/antibiotic cycle is a prime example of how conventional medicine fails to consider the root causes of a compromised immune system, thereby hampering full recovery.

Vaccinations

Vaccination—the controversial process of injecting *pathogenic* viruses and bacteria, heavy metals (e.g., mercury and aluminum), dead animal tissue, chemical preservatives, and other highly toxic substances into the bloodstream to create *synthetic* immunity—should be questioned by every concerned parent. Numerous medical doctors, natural doctors, researchers, videos, books, articles, and lawsuits have detailed the horrors of crippling conditions (temporary or permanent)—including sudden infant death syndrome (SIDS), autism, brain damage, neurological disorders, paralysis, leukemia, shock, screaming episodes, and persistent crying, to name a few—caused by subjecting the fragile immune systems of children to poison. The conventional medical paradigm (including pharmaceutical companies, medical schools, and their doctor agents backed by governmental mandates) tells us that the body requires unnatural stimulation in order to create resistance to infectious diseases. Many researchers and medical practitioners say that claim doesn't hold up to scrutiny.

The vaccination industry is a multibillion dollar a year business that facilitated a government-mandated vaccination program, even though another solution exists for disease control: natural immunity. Most diseases that have been reduced or nearly eliminated have been reined in because of better sanitation and health practices, not vaccinations; and in most cases, vaccination began *after* the incidences of disease had *already* dramatically dropped. Meanwhile, a multitude of studies show that vaccinated people have had higher incidences of the diseases they were vaccinated against than their non-vaccinated peers within the same geographical location/group.

The vaccination process itself—whereby artificial and highly toxic substances are introduced into the blood—bypasses the normal route of entry for pathogens (the gut, lungs or skin). This unnatural process not only fails to activate other required immune-building factors besides the building of antibodies, but can also contribute to the overall disintegration of the immune system (which may lead to a variety of sicknesses). For example, the synthetic immunity created by vaccination has a reinfection chance of eighty percent, whereas when immunity to a disease is acquired naturally, the possibility of reinfection is only about three percent.[3] Furthermore, numerous studies have concluded that a healthy body with a healthy immune system will *fully recover* from "dreaded" childhood diseases, even polio (renamed *aseptic meningitis* after polio vaccination began).[4]

Our bodies—including those of our children—are designed, by nature, to overcome any disease or condition, provided that the immune system is operating correctly and that our basic health is good. The bacteria and viruses that we fear are only doing their job: decomposing cells that no longer function properly. When mumps, measles, polio, or any other disease grabs hold, the body will overcome the symptoms with dispatch and create even stronger immunity. Most people do not realize this because the conventional medical paradigm continues to be disease-oriented rather than health-oriented. It's very difficult for us to throw out a paradigm or belief system into which we have been indoctrinated.

Australian researcher Viera Scheibner, PhD, in her book *Vaccination: The Medical Assault on the Immune System* (Minerva Books, 1993), writes:

> An extensive study of medical literature reveals that there is no evidence whatsoever of the ability of vaccines to prevent any diseases. To the contrary, there is a great wealth of evidence (direct and indirect) that they cause serious side effects...Immunisations, including those practiced on babies, not only did not prevent any infectious diseases, they caused more suffering and more deaths than has any other human activity in the entire history of medical intervention. It will be decades before the mopping-up after the disasters caused by childhood vaccination will be completed. All vaccinations should cease forthwith and all victims of side-effects should be appropriately compensated.[5]

Natural immunity is achieved by: avoiding refined sugar (which destroys the immune system and leaches minerals) and fluoride (which attacks the immune and endocrine systems and prevents certain enzymes from functioning); avoiding toxic food (foods grown with toxic pesticides and packaged with and in toxic chemicals); detoxification (colon cleansing and full body detoxification of heavy metals and other pathogens); eating whole, organic raw foods; consuming nutrient dense, whole food supplements; and getting exercise and sunlight. In short, taking responsibility for your health (and your children's health) by living more naturally, as nature intended.

In her book, *Immunization: The Reality Behind the Myth* (Greenwood Press, 1995), Walene James discusses the dangers and horrors of vaccination and how to build natural immunity. *Immunization* is characterized by clear detail and impeccable research: James cites hundreds of studies, doctors, and researchers to explain why and how vaccines (for polio, DPT, mumps, measles, rubella, rabbis, or tetanus) can be extremely dangerous to children; the *deliberate manipulation* of statistical data to suggest that vaccines have reduced diseases; why their purported effectiveness is highly questionable; why "diseases" are actually a product of a compromised health condition and not the other way around; why Vitamin C and an alkaline condition prevents or cures diseases (most of our bodies are acidic due to improper diet); how indigenous people around the world developed diseases only *after* they adopted our highly processed food diets; and the steps to take to develop natural immunity (through natural living). This is very helpful information for parents even remotely interested in why they should avoid the vaccine paradigm and therefore prevent the risk of permanent, vaccine-induced damage to their children.[6]

The Conventional Medicine Fallacy

The conventional medicine paradigm—based on "fighting" disease and symptom management—is fundamentally flawed. The germs (bacteria and viruses) that cause disease are around us at all times (in lesser and greater degrees). ***Simply stated, we get sick when we are not in optimum health and the immune system is not functioning properly.*** Symptoms of illness indicate imbalance in our body. Drugs may manage those symptoms, but they don't correct the underlying root causes of their appearance. Therefore, rather than identifying symptoms (with their corresponding medical names or labels) and managing those symptoms with drugs, a healthier, more natural, and more effective solution is to first understand what types of imbalances in the body are root causes of those symptoms, then work to correct those imbalances.

Chapter 4
Why Ritalin Isn't the Answer

Ritalin—and the newer Concerta (time-released Ritalin)—is an am-phetamine-like drug. It unnaturally increases the speed at which a child can deal with external stimuli (sight, sound, touch, smell, and cognitive information) by forcing faster processing through that child's weak and disorganized neural systems. Though it may appear as though the child is functioning normally, the drug may in fact be doing actual damage: For the symptoms of ADD/ADHD to exist in the first place, the child's neural pathways likely are in a disorganized and/or compromised state. To rush information through these pathways at an accelerated pace is to further tax a debilitated system.

Ritalin (methylphenidate) has been classified by the U.S. Drug Enforcement Administration (DEA) as a Schedule II drug, along with cocaine, morphine, methamphetamines, opium, and barbiturates. Chemically, it most closely resembles cocaine, which may explain some of the more disturbing facts associated with it.[1]

A study conducted at the University of Berkeley (one of the few long-term studies conducted in regard to Ritalin use) concluded that Ritalin tends to act as a "gateway" drug. The study, which followed 500 children over the course of 26 years, found that Ritalin "makes the brain more susceptible to the addictive power of cocaine and therefore, doubles the risk of abuse."[2] A similar study, documented by Richard DeGrand-pre in his book *Ritalin Nation* (W.W. Norton & Co., 1999), showed that when given the option of choosing between Ritalin or cocaine, the majority of laboratory monkeys did not show a preference for one or the other—though some preferred Ritalin, which has a slower "let down" period than cocaine. Given the drug's proven similarity to cocaine, it's no wonder that in 1995, the DEA warned that Ritalin and other methylphe-nidate-based drugs were being crushed and snorted.[3]

The agency further noted that methylphenidate "ranks in the top 10 most frequently reported controlled pharmaceuticals stolen from licensed handlers."[4] But most kids don't have to steal it. They can buy it, for an average of $7 a pill.[5] In fact, recreational use of this drug has increased along with its prescription rate. The DEA reported a sixteen percent rise in Ritalin abuse from 1992 to 1995, while the Drug Abuse Warning Net-work (DAWN) states that "the sky-rocketing use of Ritalin represents the greatest increase in drugs associated with abuse, and causes the highest number of suicides and emergency room admissions."

International Journal of the Addictions lists over 100 adverse reactions to Ritalin, including paranoid psychosis, terror, and paranoid delusions. It's no surprise that much of the school violence our nation has witnessed over the past decade has been instigated by teens who were being pre-scribed Ritalin or similar psychotropic drugs. Often, a fluctuation in dose precipitates such an episode.

Aside from such adverse reactions, Ritalin also has numerous po-tential side effects, many resembling those of cocaine's: nervousness, in-somnia, blood-pressure fluctuations, dizziness, loss of appetite, motor tics, depression, and headaches. Withdrawal symptoms are also strik-ingly similar: fatigue, disturbed sleep, depression, psychosis, and suicide.[6] Other adverse reactions to Ritalin include hallucinations and seizures, as noted on the manufacturer's insert.

What about the effects on a child's self-esteem (the reason most teachers encourage parents to consider the drug)? By forcing children to be dependent on a drug, we are telling them that they are incapable of functioning without it. Though many psychiatrists attribute feelings of isolation and loneliness to untreated cases of attention disorders, many children report such feelings as a result of taking medication.

According to a National Institutes of Health consensus statement,

"[A]n independent diagnostic test for ADHD does not exist,"[7] which makes diagnosing it questionable in the first place and prescribing medication for it more or less a crapshoot. Additionally, symptoms of attention disorders can be easily confused with, among other things, seizure disorders, certain learning disabilities, clinical depression, bipolar disorder, and post-traumatic stress disorder. Giving medication to a child suffering from one of these can all but muzzle a cry for help—one of the observable characteristics of Ritalin is that it makes the children taking it much more compliant.

It is a natural parental instinct to want children to succeed and to be accepted, even if that means conforming to preset social norms. Lawrence Diller, MD, author of the bestselling book *Running on Ritalin* (Bantam, 1999), has written that "Ritalin will help round and octagonal peg kids fit into rather rigid square educational holes."

But research shows that improved classroom performance is the only positive short-term outcome of Ritalin use. As Richard DeGrandpre wrote in a recent article, "Dozens of objective studies have assessed the long-term effectiveness of stimulants on children's academic performance, social development, and self-control. None has shown them to be effective for anything but controlling the kids' behavior—an effect that vanishes once the drug wears off."[8]

Because of its short-term effect and its only positive attribute being that the child's classroom behavior improves, many doctors and educators are beginning to consider Ritalin not much more than a performance pill. Other medications have been developed and marketed to attempt to enhance children's, and adults', abilities to sustain focused attention. Yet Concerta, Adderall, Adderall XR, Cylert, Strattera, Dexedrine, and other drugs are also gaining recognition for their deleterious side effects, ranging from strokes, to increased incidence of suicide in children and adolescents, to even death. Strattera can cause liver damage, upset stomach, decreased appetite, nausea or vomiting, tiredness, dizziness, and mood swings.[9]

There is growing concern that ADD and ADHD are just convenient labels to throw over those whose learning styles are perhaps more hands-on and activity-oriented than others. Clearly, there are children who exhibit behavioral problems, but whether these problems are truly pathological, and not a valid response to an increasingly information-addled society, is at the ethical crux of the debate over Ritalin and other psychotropic medications used to increase attention span for school and work-related tasks.[10]

In the words of Peter Breggin, MD, a leading critic against prescribing medication to treat attention disorders: "We are the first adults to handle the generation gap through the wholesale drugging of our children. We may be guaranteeing that future generations will be relatively devoid of people who think critically, raise painful questions, generate productive conflicts, or lead us to new spiritual or political insights."[11]

Many children who are intellectually gifted also display some or all of what are considered to be traits of ADD/ADHD. Throughout history, there have been stories of the genius or inventor who was mistaken as a problem child. But is taking a drug like Ritalin going to affect a child's mind permanently, or if the child is gifted, "dumb" him down to a level of normality? We don't know. We do know that long-term stimulant abuse negatively affects the physical structure of the brain, causing cortical atrophy (i.e., brain deterioration)."[12]

If the only benefit a child may gain from taking Ritalin is better performance in the classroom, while the negative side effects and possible adverse reactions are greatly disproportionate, who stands to gain from the sale of these drugs?

Clearly, the overworked teacher—whose classroom is twice the size it should be—breathes a sigh of relief when the boy who was loudly interrupting and bouncing in and out of his seat last week now sits quietly and pays attention because he's taken his pill. And the parents of the girl who refused to do her homework and responded defiantly to every request are overjoyed when she sits down to study unprompted and obsequiously does what she's told. But behavioral improvements wear off when the drug is out of the child's system; the efficacy (and dangers) of long-term use of these medications is unknown; and, eventually, children, parents, and teachers will be forced to confront the repercussions of delaying the development of internal coping mechanisms in lieu of a chemical straitjacket.

It seems that pharmaceutical companies are the big winners here. Through alliances with supposedly unbiased organizations such as Children and Adults with Attention Deficit Hyperactivity Disorder (CHADD), drug manufacturers have created additional avenues for hyping their products. It was recently discovered that over the course of a few years CHADD had received over $1 million from Novartis, the maker of Ritalin.[13]

"I've been offered $100 to sit and listen to someone talk about ADHD, funded by Adderall, for fifteen minutes…" Lawrence Diller has said.[14] And the marketing of these drugs doesn't stop with physicians, "parent groups," or researchers: drug companies are now going straight to the consumer.

In a recent issue of *Parade Magazine*, a full-page ad celebrates "[p]utting control of your child's ADHD right where it belongs…in your hands." The beneficent company so concerned with your child's well-being is Shire US Inc., "Your ADHD Support Company." Nowhere does the ad mention that Shire US Inc. is part of the international pharmaceutical company Shire—which manufactures the ADHD drugs Adderall and Adderall XR.

As the consumption of psychotropic drugs reaches an all-time high, few of us seem willing to question why. However, because the pharmaceutical empires producing these drugs are big businesses that must turn hefty profits in order to survive, we not only have a right but a responsibility to question their motives. In no area is this questioning more important than in the realm of our children's health.

The coming chapters will show you how the symptoms of ADD/ ADHD can be alleviated and eradicated through non-drug methods. Giving Ritalin or any other stimulant or psychotropic drug to a child masks the actual health problems he or she is experiencing—and postpones improvement of neurological functioning. Parents, doctors, and teachers should realize that, almost invariably, *when children "misbehave" they are actually trying to communicate to us that something is wrong.* An inability to sit still and listen, to pay attention, or to follow through with things *indicates that something in the brain and the nervous system in general is not working properly.* Wouldn't it be better to figure out what isn't working properly in the brain, then permanently fix the problem, rather than just manage symptoms with toxic drugs? This book shows you how.

Chapter 5
Attentional Priority Disorder,
Not Attention Deficit Disorder

The link between neurological challenges and attention disorders has been studied and explained extensively by Judith Bluestone, founder of The HANDLE® Institute, headquartered in Seattle, Washington.[1] HANDLE (an acronym for Holistic Approach to Neurodevelopment and Learning Efficiency) considers labels such as ADD or ADHD to be limiting and impractical. Bluestone acknowledges that broad diagnostic terms may serve the purpose of providing "a sort of shorthand with which to discuss clusters of symptoms." That said, Bluestone adds, "No one yet knows how to treat a label."[2]

Not only are labels like ADD and ADHD limiting, they may not accurately reflect the experiences of a child diagnosed with these conditions: Bluestone and HANDLE contend that there is no such thing as an attention "deficit." As Bluestone says, "Everyone is always attending to something." The question is to what. The ability to manage sights, sounds, physical sensations, and other stimuli taken in by the senses is often compromised in children diagnosed with ADD/ADHD. Their subsequent struggle to feel at ease in their surroundings and even in their own skin absorbs their attention—and takes priority over staying in their seat, heeding directions, or remaining focused on schoolwork. Consequently, Bluestone has reclassified the symptoms associated with ADD/ADHD as **Attentional Priority Disorder**, a term that is less limiting yet more representative of the conditions behind attention disorders.

Children with attention disorders may have a poor sense of equilibrium and movement, or perhaps they are highly sensitive to sights, sounds, or tactile sensations. They become unable to respond to a teacher's instructions amid the glare of fluorescent lights, the rumbling of the copy machine, another student's tapping foot, the sensation of clothing against the skin, or the feeling of being unbalanced and precariously situated in space. For the ADD/ADHD-labeled child, such stimuli enter his or her consciousness at the same priority level, *causing sensory overload* and a consequential "shut down."

An attention disorder results from disorganization in the neurological systems that provide information to the brain (via vision, hearing, or other senses). The child is paying attention to certain sights, sounds, or other information because doing so seems necessary to ensure his or her feelings of safety and security—after all, our first response is always for survival. Unfortunately, to others this may look like the child is not "paying attention." *But the child's behavior is a direct response to sensory overload, the result of neurological dysfunction.*

Behavior and the Brain

There are many neurological systems that are part of the central nervous system and provide information to the brain, including the vestibular system (the very important and complex inner-ear system that affects and supports numerous other neurological systems), olfaction (smell), gustation (taste), tactility (touch), muscle tone (the muscles' readiness to respond to stimuli), kinesthesia (one's awareness of movement), proprioception (the unconscious awareness of the dynamic sense of body in space), oral-motor function, audition, visual functions (including eye teaming and tracking), differentiation, laterality, and interhemispheric integration. All of these systems must work properly, and together, in order for a person to function "normally." Diagnosis of ADD/ADHD, Asperger's syndrome, Tourette's syndrome, dyslexia, autism, and other neurological disorders may occur depending on 1) which of these neurological systems is compromised or not connecting efficiently to other systems and 2) the severity of the weakness within any given neurological system(s) or interaction of systems. Neural pathways in the brain and other organs and systems transmit information—gathered by the systems enumerated above (e.g., vision, hearing, smell, touch, taste, muscle tension, equilibrium, and body-in-space) and other visceral systems as well—through a variety of processing systems. These systems interface our past (memory), present (sensory), and future (intention and aspiration) to give us appropriate plans for action, be it speech, reasoning, movement, refrainment from action, reading, writing, or another response. When the neural pathways become disorganized and/or are underdeveloped and thin, messages tend to be transmitted at a sluggish pace, causing "bottlenecks" and sensory overload.[3]

Messages may subsequently be discarded because they haven't received the repeated transmissions required to support the development of connective neural pathways. Or the child may still be processing the first message when new messages come along, causing confusion.[4] The brain is then susceptible to becoming overwhelmed by normal sensory input, resulting in a "shut down" of some of the neural systems. This shut down may cause the outbursts and emotional meltdowns sometimes seen in children suffering from ADD/ADHD—they are acting out in anger and frustration over not being able to concentrate on, comprehend, and respond appropriately to the tasks at hand. This is frequently the result of a compromised vestibular system (inner ear) that is not able to simultaneously support vision, hearing, movement, and a sense of body-in-space, all of which are necessary in order first to feel safe and secure, and then to respond appropriately to a task in a reasonable amount of time. Additionally, overstimulation of a hypersensitive and/or disorganized system may feel like an assault, in which case the child may respond reactively or even reflexively, rather than responsively.

Outer Behavior, Inner Challenges

Watching a child's outer behavior can offer insight into his or her inner neurological challenges, if you know what to look for. For example, the child who *looks away when you talk to her* may need to reduce visual overload so she can listen to you. The child who *slumps down in his chair* may be exhibiting that he has low muscle tone, and until he relaxes all his muscles he may not be able to pay attention. The child who *wants to wear loose clothing* may be telling us that he has tactile issues and is bothered by the feel of cloth on his body; until his tactile issues are resolved, he won't be able to pay attention to anything else. The child who *wears a visor* may need to keep the high frequency flickering fluorescent light from assaulting her visual system so she can pay attention. The child *drumming with the pencil or constantly moving around* may be telling us that her inner ear isn't working properly, and she must move to keep the vestibular system energized in order to pay attention. Until a child (or an adult) can attend to the neurological challenges dictated by her unique set of circumstances, *she won't be able to pay attention to what others want her to attend to.*

Survival and Solutions

"If a situation is causing us distress," Bluestone says, "we will engage in self-protective behaviors. All of us protect ourselves in the areas of our greatest vulnerability." Safety and survival must be our highest priority so we will live to see another day. Children with Attentional Priority Disorder have varying areas of vulnerability, which often surface via strange or disruptive behaviors—an unconscious attempt to sift through the onslaught of information that seems to be bombarding them from all sides. Through HANDLE methodologies, neurologically challenged children can become capable of prioritizing their attention and controlling their behavior; permanently, and without drugs, once the health of the vestibular system and other neural pathways and systems are restored.

The "organized movement" activities that HANDLE has developed engage these neural pathways and systems, thereby strengthening them: an activity might involve hopping on one leg and then the other in a certain pattern, thus engaging the vestibular system, which affects balance, as well as neurological systems relevant to muscle tone, muscle differentiation, and use of the brain's left and right hemispheres. These exercises' targeted use of compromised neurological pathways and systems will enhance and repair them—and ultimately improve neurological functioning.

Like all natural or alternative health solutions, the HANDLE approach addresses the causes of a problem instead of merely treating symptoms. The next 2 chapters will explore the varied possible reasons that neurological systems can be compromised to begin with and then the many available non-drug solutions are discussed.

Chapter 6
Possible Causes of
Neurological Disorders

As noted in Chapter 5, attention disorders are the consequence of weaknesses in neurological systems. These weaknesses may have occurred before, during, or after birth. They can be the result of any number of overlapping causes, each with varying degrees of significance. And there can be dozens of internal and/or external factors that contribute—or that *have* contributed—to each underlying cause.

If you understand the constellation of possible causes behind neurological weakness, you can help reverse those causes—and improve your child's neurological functioning.

This chapter lists and describes many factors that may give way to poor health and subsequent neurological weakness: toxic lifestyles, inadequate nutrition, dairy consumption, candida growth, fluoride toxicity, heavy metals (and mercury amalgam fillings), prenatal and postnatal conditions, seizures, and the dangerous chemicals that infiltrate all aspects of our daily lives.

The brain is particularly susceptible to neurological malfunction when 1) highly toxic chemicals or heavy metals have crossed the blood/brain barrier and/or 2) the brain does not receive adequate nutrition, especially amino acids and omega-3 fatty acids. (A lack of minerals and vitamins also significantly limit or compromise brain function.) Inadequate nutrition and brain poisoning can be easily traced to the toxic food we eat daily, while heavy metals such as mercury and aluminum can get into the brain from vaccinations and other sources. Other dangerous chemicals found in carpet, varnishes, paint, toxic cleaning products and household goods enter the brain through inhalation or skin contact.

While reading, keep in mind that the information presented here isn't meant to induce blame or guilt for past decisions or behaviors, which were likely carried out with the best of intentions and available knowledge. Rather, this chapter, like the rest of the book, exists to help you create a future of smart, healthy choices that improve neurological functioning and overall well-being.

The Toxic Lifestyle (and the Body-Brain Connection)

Poor general health (characterized by low energy, frequent or chronic sickness, irritability, allergies, constant runny nose, and other conditions) is a sign that the body is not working optimally. And if the body as a whole is not working optimally, then brain function is likely to be deficient. The first step toward healing neurological disorders—and, consequently, attention disorders—is to *actively work on healing the body as a whole*. Avoiding a toxic lifestyle and adopting a natural living lifestyle (discussed in Chapter 7) is the best possible course of action for total body healing.

The toxic lifestyle significantly contributes to poor health and neurological disorders. Check out this list of toxic "don'ts" (some of which this or other chapters discuss in greater detail):

- Eating fast food.
- Eating foods grown with pesticides and herbicides.
- Eating foods preserved, colored, and flavored with synthetic chemicals.
- Eating nutritionally stripped foods.
- Eating foods with high sugar content.
- Eating genetically modified and irradiated foods.
- Eating conventional meat (laced with antibiotics, synthetic growth hormones, tranquilizers, pesticides, and diseased animal parts).
- Consuming cow dairy products—milk, cheese and yogurt (laced with antibiotics, synthetic growth hormones, tranquilizers, pesti-

cides, and diseased animal parts).
- Using antibiotics.
- Using toxic household cleaners.
- Using skin care and body products made from synthetic chemicals.
- Drinking chlorinated and fluoridated water.
- Not exercising.
- Not colon cleansing and detoxifying the body on a regular basis.
- Turning one's health responsibility over to insurance companies, HMOs, and conventional (allopathic) medical doctors.
- Being vaccinated with pathogenic bacteria and deadly heavy metals.
- Using prescription drugs to manage and mask the symptoms of unbalanced body chemistry.
- Believing that the use of prescription drugs is the only option available.
- Believing doctors and the media when they say that neurological disorders and diseases, such as cancer, are incurable.
- Believing the mainstream media without investigation.
- Believing the lie that healing isn't possible.

In short, toxic living is a *lifestyle choice*—encouraged by multinational corporations, governmental agencies, medical authorities, and the media. It deprives the body of required nutrition, feeds us potentially harmful chemicals, and uses drugs to manage resultant conditions, creating even more toxicity and disease. Believing in and following this synthetically based paradigm is the primary reason for disease and neurological disorders.

The Wrong Diet
The all-pervasive, ongoing, deliberate manipulation of our food supply—from the farm to the shelf, and at every step in between—is the single greatest contributor to poor health. Without a doubt, the contamination of our food with synthetic chemicals (pesticides, herbicides, heavy metals, preservatives, food dyes, stabilizers, artificial flavorings, synthetic vitamins, growth hormones, tranquilizers, antibiotics, and the like) combined with production techniques that decimate the intrinsic nutritional value of raw food (genetic engineering, irradiation, high-temperature processing, hydrogenation, and so on) is a root cause of poor health. Our

bodies and brains are not designed by nature to operate on nutritionally stripped, chemically laden food day in and day out. Daily intake of microscopically small doses of toxins (and massive doses of toxins, such as from vaccinations) contributes dramatically to ill health—and therefore reduced brain function. For more information on the dangers of conventional food, read Chapter 2 of my book *The Beginner's Guide to Natural Living*, pages 33–67.

Dairy Products[1]

Why are so many children allergic to cow's milk? Because they don't need it—not because there is something wrong with them. The revered pediatrician Benjamin Spock warned that "cow's milk...has definite faults for some babies. It causes allergies, indigestion, and contributes to some cases of childhood diabetes." Frank A. Oski, former director of pediatrics at Johns Hopkins University, bluntly stated: "There's no reason to drink cow's milk *at any time in your life*. It was designed for calves, not humans, and we should all stop drinking it today" (italics mine).

The intestines of some babies wind up bleeding after cow's milk has been consumed, resulting in iron loss. After age four, many children become lactose intolerant. For these children, milk proteins seep into the immune system and can result in chronic runny noses, sore throats, hoarseness, bronchitis, and recurring ear infections—the symptoms of "milk allergies." Some children's bodies react to cow's milk protein as a foreign substance, then produce high levels of antibodies in fending it off. These antibodies also destroy the cells that produce insulin in the pancreas, possibly paving the path toward diabetes.

Human breast milk is approximately five and a half percent protein, designed to double an infant's birth weight in about 180 days. Cow's milk, on the other hand, is about *fifteen* percent protein—it's meant to double the weight of a calf in just forty-seven days. Human babies who are fed cow's milk may only digest about half of the protein, straining their developing kidneys. When cow's milk mixes with an infant's digestive juices in the stomach, large curds develop because of the casein content, and that can lead to health problems. Whereas human milk is sterile, cow's milk is not, and feeding it to infants can introduce harmful organisms to a weak immune system. There's more saturated fat as well, which increases cholesterol in the infant. Pasteurization of cow's milk kills some harmful microorganisms, but it also destroys important lactobacillus bacteria and vitamins, which are normally found in human breast milk. Pasteurization also creates long-chain fatty acids that are more difficult for the intestinal tract to process. The high protein content of milk produces an acidic environment in the body. To correct the acidic environment, the body will withdraw calcium from the bones—which are alkaline—to bring the PH level back in balance. Although dairy is high in calcium, it can't be fully assimilated because of the high phosphorous content—calcium absorption occurs when there is a low phosphorous to high calcium ratio. The excess calcium floating in the blood, from the bones and from the milk, is then filtered through the kidneys, precipitating kidney stones later in life.

In addition to these issues, we also get the chemical stew from the aggressive agricultural practices found in the dairy industry. Dairy cows are unnaturally kept pregnant 24/7 to produce twenty times their normal amount of milk. They are housed in unsanitary conditions (often on conveyer belts). This leads to disease of the udder and to the dairy cows in general (including bovine leukemia, found in eighty-nine percent of dairy cows). Under these conditions, a cow's average lifespan drops from twenty years to about four. Antibiotics are used to slow disease, tranquilizers are used to calm frayed nerves, and artificial growth hormones are injected to increase milk production. The cows' feed is laden with pesticide and herbicide residue and other chemicals. Remember—what cows consume, we consume too.

Candida Overgrowth
Candida albicans is a type of parasitic yeast-like fungus that inhabits the intestines, genital region, mouth, esophagus, throat, and even the brain. Ordinarily, candida lives uneventfully in our intestinal tract and is "checked" by other microorganisms and friendly bacteria. But candida will multiply out of control and cause a host of health problems if these friendly bacteria are destroyed and/or the immune system is compromised—often a consequence of exposure to mercury or certain drugs, including antibiotics.

Symptoms of candida overgrowth include nasal congestion and discharge, nasal itching, blisters in the mouth, abdominal pain, bloating, heartburn, constipation, diarrhea, vaginal discharge or burning, frequent urination, burning on urination, and bladder infections. Oral thrush, jock itch, and athlete's foot are all consequences of candida overgrowth, as are other ongoing health problems. If the immune system remains weak long enough, candida can spread to all parts of the body and cause an additional plethora of health woes, including mood swings, anxiety, and difficulty concentrating. People who have candida infections also often have food allergies. And, very importantly, *candida overgrowth can inhibit proper assimilation of nutrients, including essential amino acids*,[2] which will adversely affect brain function.

Consuming foods high in sugar, yeast, or simple carbohydrates can lead to candida overgrowth, as can antibiotics if they are used frequently. A weakened immune system also allows candida to proliferate—so build the immune system with a natural living lifestyle (see Chapter 7) to reduce candida overgrowth. Other ways of controlling candida include eliminating processed foods and consuming ample amounts of acidophilus and other friendly bacteria (such as the Bio-K brand found in natural food stores). A visit to a natural doctor, such as a naturopathic physician, is also advised.

Fluoride

Part of the controversy about fluoride results from confusion over calcium fluoride, used in the original tooth decay-prevention tests, and sodium fluoride, a highly toxic industrial waste product from the phosphate fertilizer industry. Unfortunately, it's sodium fluoride that's added to city water supplies.[3] Approximately sixty-seven percent of American cities fluoridate municipal water.

Sodium fluoride kills many of your bodies' beneficial enzymes. It also attacks the hypothalamus gland (which regulates hunger, thirst, body temperature, and one's sense of safety and comfort). Furthermore, over-ingestion of fluoride impairs the thyroid gland, which regulates metabolism. (Could this contribute to the alarming rate of obesity in the United States?)

Additionally, sodium fluoride may weaken bones (a condition called skeletal fluorosis), and can cause dental fluorosis in children.[4] Dental fluorosis, a mineralization disorder of the teeth that degrades the enamel, is an irreversible condition caused by excessive ingestion of fluoride during the tooth-forming years.

Sodium fluoride is also a very powerful central nervous system toxin that can adversely affect human brain functioning and diminish IQ, even at low doses.[5]

Contrary to the propaganda we hear in the media, the largest survey ever done on tooth decay, conducted by the National Institute of Dental Research, found *no* difference in tooth decay between fluoridated and nonfluoridated communities in the United States, as measured in terms of decayed, missing, and filled teeth.[6] Word about fluoridated water's risks and ineffectiveness may be getting out: Over eighty U.S. cities have rejected fluoridation since 1996. (Europe has almost unanimously rejected it—only two percent of the entire continent allows water fluoridation.)

If your community's water supply is fluoridated, it's best to avoid drinking tap water unless a filter is used to remove the fluoride. See www.custompure.com for high-quality water filters. For more information on fluoride dangers, visit the Fluoride Action Network's Web site at www.fluoridealert.org.

Mercury Poisoning

Mercury is such a deadly substance that even minimal exposure, as little as a drop on your hand, can prove fatal. It's the second most toxic element after plutonium and is estimated to be 500 to 1,000 times more toxic than lead. This heavy metal burrows deep into the cells of the brain and other organs and can lead to serious central nervous system damage and crippling neurological disorders. It is a neurotoxin[7] that acts directly on the tissues of the central nervous system. Mercury is even more neurotoxic than lead, cadmium, or arsenic.[8] Unfortunately, it is used in vaccines and amalgam fillings, both widespread treatments that are designed to improve our health—and that may make us sick.

Mercury and Vaccines

Numerous studies indicate that the behavioral and psychological disposition of children diagnosed with autism is *nearly identical* to people who have confirmed *mercury poisoning*.[9] Often, children diagnosed with autism began to show the symptoms shortly after vaccination. Many vaccines are (still) preserved with mercury, and children can easily exceed the U.S. Environmental Protection Agency's (EPA) recommended dose of "allowable" mercury exposure through vaccination. (For an in-depth and concise overview on the direct link between mercury poisoning and autism symptoms and other neurological disorders, visit Generation Rescue at www.generationrescue.org.)

Though not all children vaccinated exhibit signs of autism, many do show other neurological processing difficulties or are diagnosed with ADD/ADHD, dyslexia, and other problems that can be linked, in part, to mercury poisoning.

Amalgam Fillings
Mercury amalgam ("silver") fillings contain about fifty percent mercury, along with silver, tin, and zinc. Conventional dental authorities allege that mercury is "locked" into the filling because the atomic structure of mercury is "bound" to the silver, rendering the state of the mercury biologically inactive. However, studies have shown that mercury vapor escapes on a regular basis and is absorbed by the rest of the body. This vapor release increases while eating or drinking hot foods and liquids, during chewing (friction releases the vapor), or if an amalgam filling is located next to a tooth that has been restored with gold or other metals. Mercury vapor released from amalgam fillings has been shown to accumulate in organs, the brain, fetal tissue, and maternal milk. This low-level (but continuous) mercury exposure can cause mercury poisoning, which will produce a variety of health problems, including neurological disorders. (Tremors are a common indicator of mercury neurotoxicity.)

If you decide to have amalgam fillings removed, choose an experienced *holistic* dentist who follows specific protocols that will protect you against mercury exposure during the removal process. Sudden intense introduction of vaporous mercury that may occur during improper removal of fillings can be more dangerous than keeping the fillings in your teeth.

When you take into consideration the amount of mercury exposure mothers receive from mercury amalgam fillings and fish consumption, combined with what children receive because of vaccinations and their *own* mercury amalgam fillings and fish consumption, there shouldn't be any surprise at all why we now face an epidemic of neurologically challenged children. (And that's just taking into account mercury exposure *without* including the other toxic chemicals that afflict us.)

Other Heavy Metal Poisoning

Heavy metal poisoning is the toxic accumulation of heavy metals—such as mercury, lead, cadmium, and arsenic—in the soft tissues of the body. Toxic heavy metals will displace essential minerals, like zinc, copper, magnesium, and calcium, and can cause cognitive and behavioral problems or even mental retardation. Lead, cadmium, and arsenic can enter the body through environmental factors (e.g., lead paint or polluted dirt) or through the diet. In fact, extremely toxic industrial waste is legally "recycled" into the nation's fertilizer supply, which is dumped into our food supply.[10]

Heavy metals can easily accumulate in the brain and cause neurological problems because they are so widespread in our diet and environment. Adopting a natural living lifestyle significantly reduces this potential exposure.

Prenatal and Postnatal Risks

During pregnancy, the overall toxicity level and nutritional level of the mother will directly affect fetal brain development. Physical and emotional stress can further obstruct the normal, healthy functioning of a developing brain by suppressing the immune system. A mother's lack of movement during pregnancy (because of watching TV, working at the computer, mandatory bed rest, and so forth) may impair proper fetal neurological development. On the other hand, too much movement may create a stressful environment for the fetus, also impairing neurological development.

A brain that fails to grow to normal size in utero due to malnutrition, prescription drugs, nicotine, or harmful intoxicants—such as alcohol or cocaine—can contribute to neurological disorders. Ultrasound, frequently used to monitor the health of the developing fetus and also to ascertain the sex of the fetus for curious parents, produces sound waves that stress the developing vestibular system.

The delivery process itself may cause problems if the baby passes too quickly or not quickly enough through the birth canal, or if the baby is delivered by Caesarean section. Head trauma caused either during the birthing process (by prolonged labor, forceps delivery, or suction) and/or from an accidental injury is a potential cause of neurological disorders—such trauma can result in structural damage to the brain, as well as damage to the vestibular system *and* other neural pathways. Babies delivered in a hospital setting with the best of intentions and care are brought into the world in a bright, reflective, possibly noisy environment filled with numerous and noxious odors—then they're quickly scrubbed clean of the slimy coating that is meant to protect them from such an abrupt change of environment. Such experiences can increase stress on the infant, particularly if its systems are already vulnerable.

After birth, coordinated activity—including crawling—helps to organize the neural pathways in the brain (use of "baby walkers" should therefore be avoided). And conversely, inactivity (e.g., watching TV or playing video games) and/or a lack of *coordinated* physical activity can significantly limit the proper growth and function of neurological systems. Ear infections can *severely affect vestibular system function*, which in turn can significantly reduce or otherwise affect overall neurological processing ability. People diagnosed with ADD/ADHD often have had recurrent ear infections. The correlation between ear infections and decreased neurological functioning is frequently overlooked—if there are/ were recurrent ear infections, then vestibular system damage should be suspected.

Brain Seizures

A higher than usual incidence of seizures is seen in people with mental retardation and a variety of other neurobehavioral disorders, such as autism, Tourette's syndrome, attention disorders, and reactive attachment disorder (RAD). A child who "spaces out" on a regular basis—mimicking ADD/ADHD—may be experiencing brain seizures, evidencing a seizure disorder rather than an attention deficit. An EEG/QEEG neurological assessment can identify whether seizures are in fact taking place. These tests become even more important if stimulant medication—which can induce brain seizures—is being taken to address ADD/ADHD.

EEG is the abbreviation for electroencephalography, meaning the process of detecting and recording brainwaves. The brainwaves are recorded with sensors placed on the scalp. The "Q" in QEEG refers to the "quantitative analysis" of the EEG recording. QEEGs, developed in the 1970's and 80's, use computerized statistical and analytical techniques, whereas the EEG does not. The QEEG procedure is an extension of (not a substitute for) clinical EEG testing; it is also complementary to tests such as the MRI, which image brain structure, not function.

The EEG/QEEG is a measure of brain function or activity. It measures changes in patterns of brain function over short periods of time. This type of analysis is completely noninvasive, cost effective, and does not involve exposure to radioactive agents.

The EEG has been used in neurology, psychiatry, and other fields of medicine since the 1950's. One of its first uses was to identify periods of brainwave activity during sleep, even when the study subject appeared quiet and motionless. (If the subject was awakened during this time, he often reported that he had been dreaming.) EEGs, along with QEEGs, continue to be used in peeking "below the surface" of behavior to assess underlying brain processes. They are primarily utilized to identify brain seizures.

Often, seizures do not cause obvious convulsions, characterized by the rolling of the eyes, biting the tongue, and so forth. Convulsions are seen in "grand mal" type seizures. It is common to have seizure activity that is associated with lapse in awareness rather than convulsions. "Petit mal" seizures, as well as other types of "partial seizures," are usually accompanied by a brief loss of awareness. As noted above, the seizure event may not be recognized as a seizure and may be described as "spacing out" or "glazing over." This loss of awareness is often mistaken for inattentiveness in the classroom. It is useful to evaluate those experiences with EEG/QEEG tests, because seizures are often the culprit. These assessments allow for health practitioners to evaluate the neurological events underlying behavioral problems. They help in suggesting specific treatment interventions and monitoring changes in the nervous system produced by interventions.

Pesticides, Herbicides, and Other Chemicals
Pesticides, herbicides, and other chemical poisons that find their way into the food chain can cause numerous health problems and impair neurological functioning. Remember Agent Orange, the toxic spray used by the U.S. military in Vietnam in clearing away forests? It ultimately caused health problems for our veterans and birth defects in their children. Two of the toxic chemicals found in Agent Orange, 2,4-D and 2,4,5-T, are sprayed on land used to grow feed for livestock.[11] One of these chemicals is dioxin, used in 2,4,5-T. Even more toxic than DDT,

dioxin causes cancer, birth defects, miscarriages, and almost immediate death in lab animals at even *one part per trillion.* In 1974, Environmental Protection Agency official Dianne Courtney called dioxin "by far the most toxic chemical known to mankind."[12] *Yet dioxin is legally used on the food we eat.*

According to the Environmental Working Group (www.ewg.org):

> More than a million preschoolers consume at least fifteen pesticides a day in food, according to our latest study of government data. Some 324,000 kids age five and under exceed federal safety standards every day for just one neurotoxic insecticide, methyl parathion. Methyl parathion is the most toxic organophosphate insecticide approved for use on food. It's so toxic that the EPA's "daily" safe dose for the compound is 0.000025 milligrams per kilogram of human body weight. A 154 pound person would exceed the EPA daily dose by eating less than two one-millionths of a gram of the chemical (.002 milligrams). Some apples and peaches are so contaminated with methyl parathion that a kid can exceed the government's safe daily limits with just two bites. A 154-pound adult eating such an apple would ingest only half of the current safe daily dose, whereas it would put a forty-four pound child sixty-seven percent over his or her *"safe"* limit.[13]

Organophosphate pesticides inhibit the enzyme acetylcholinesterase, a key molecule required to permit the regeneration of acetylcholine at neuromuscular junctions and thereby control nerve-to-muscle transmission. Many organophosphorus compounds damage nerves directly, creating adverse conditions that are largely irreversible. Animal studies show that organophosphorus compounds damage the central nervous system. Neurological poisoning may take months or years to show up. Concentrated organophosphorus compounds are used to produce nerve gas, and a few drops are quickly lethal.[14] Symptoms of poisoning include stomach and intestinal cramps, vomiting, diarrhea, and "pinpoint" pupils. These pesticides change chemically as they age, becoming even more toxic.

Dozens of pesticides and herbicides used today disrupt the human endocrine system.[15] In late 1995, a multidisciplinary group of international experts (medical doctors, university scholars, environmentalists, and others) gathered in Erice, Sicily, for a work session on "Environmental Endocrine-Disrupting Chemicals: Neural, Endocrine, and Behavioral Effects."[16] The committee wrote:

> Thyroid hormones are essential for normal brain function throughout life. Interference with thyroid hormone function during development leads to abnormalities in brain and behavioral development. The eventual results of moderate to severe alterations of thyroid hormone concentrations, *particularly during fetal life*, are motor dysfunction of varying severity, including cerebral palsy, mental retardation, learning disability, attention deficit hyperactivity disorder, hydrocephalus, seizures, and other neurological abnormalities. Similarly, exposure to man-made chemicals during early development can impair motor function, spatial perception, learning, memory, auditory development, fine motor coordination, balance, and attention processes; in severe cases, mental retardation may result. Because certain PCBs and dioxins are known to impair normal thyroid function, we suspect that they *contribute to learning disabilities, including attention deficit hyperactivity disorder and other neurological abnormalities* (italics mine)."[17]

Food Additives

As if it weren't enough that toxic pesticides, herbicides, and fungicides are sprayed onto food crops, most manufacturers then lace what we eat with a cornucopia of harmful synthetic chemicals during processing. Since 1959, more than twenty-five chemical food additives have been banned because they cause cancer or other serious diseases in laboratory animals. Dozens of other additives are currently under review by the U.S. Food and Drug Administration. You might be familiar with some of these substances: food dyes, preservatives, flavorings, stabilizers, anti-mold agents, and so on. Unfortunately, our bodies can't use these chemicals; physiologically, we react to them as we would to a poison.

Disturbingly, by the time an American child is five years old, he will have consumed more than seven and a half pounds of food additives through preservatives, emulsifiers, lubricants, bleaching agents, synthetic sweeteners, flavor enhancers, and artificial colors and flavors.[18] Research has linked some synthetic additives with hyperactivity and behavioral changes—as well as with asthma (which frequently afflicts those diagnosed with ADD/ADHD), cancer, and other serious ailments.

The late Ben F. Feingold, MD, author of *Why Your Child Is Hyperactive* (Random House, 1996), was among the first medical professionals to maintain that synthetic food dyes, preservatives, and flavorings can cause severe behavioral changes in both children and adults. Feingold's research helped get some toxic synthetics banned in the United States. His pioneering work also led to the Feingold Diet for attention disorders (discussed at www.feingold.org), which eliminates all foods containing synthetic dyes and food flavorings. Also eliminated are the synthetic antioxidant preservative chemicals butylated hydroxyanisole (BHA), butylated hydroxytoluene (BHT), and tertiary butylhydroquinone (TBHQ), as well as aspirin and other salicylates (naturally occurring compounds found in some fruits, vegetables, and toiletries). Thousands of children who have followed this diet showed marked improvement in behavior—and often recovered from attention disorders because their brain chemistry was normalized.[19]

Brominated Fire Retardants

Brominated fire retardants, known as PBDEs (polybrominated diphenyl ethers), are added to everyday products, such as computers, cars, TVs, and furniture. They are persistent in the indoor environment and are also bioaccumulative, building up in people's bodies over a lifetime. Children may ingest significant amounts of toxic fire retardants from the dust found inside the house. In minute doses brominated fire retardants impair attention, learning, memory, and behavior in laboratory animals.[20]

Other sources of potential chemical contamination to children include carpet, varnishes, toxic household cleaning products, and body products with synthetic chemicals.

Our Toxic World

As you can see, we live in and ingest a toxic world—funded by megamultinational corporations and endorsed by the government. The food we eat is highly polluted, genetically modified, irradiated, stripped of nutrition, and packed full of synthetic chemicals. Unnecessary vaccinations add extremely dangerous levels of highly toxic heavy metals to the developing brains and bodies of children. Chlorine and fluoride wreak havoc on the body. Antibiotics contribute to candida growth and the destruction of the immune system. Birth trauma, sedentary lifestyles, ear infections, and other factors (besides toxicity) can contribute to neurological dysfunction. And when you put it all together, it's easy to see how diagnoses of ADD/ADHD, autism, dyslexia, and other neurological disorders manifest. Is there hope? You bet there is: the answers are found in natural living and alternative medicine.

Chapter 7
Nontoxic Solutions

To say that "everything causes cancer" may make for a piquant observation, but it's also a pessimistic one that ignores how people can enjoy healthy lives—and recover from attention disorders as well as other neurological challenges—when they adopt a natural lifestyle.

Corporations and other organizations go to great lengths to mislead you, to convince you that disorders and disease aren't caused by the food you eat and other non-genetic factors, that true healing is impossible, that you must rely on drugs and doctors to manage your health problems. *In truth, the body (including the brain), in most instances, can repair itself, when given the right conditions.* Consider the many things you can do to improve your neurological functioning and overall health:

1. Shield your body and brain from the many sources of toxin intake. It's particularly important to limit conventionally produced, synthetic-laden, nutritionally stripped food, and to consider avoiding vaccinations.
2. Detox from built-up toxins and pathogens, especially heavy metals.
3. Consume the most nutritious food available (i.e., whole, organic food) while using proper food combinations and meal-preparation techniques.

4. Take nutritional supplements for added nutrition and functional support.
5. Visit natural/alternative healing practitioners who specialize in your area of concern and promote overall health in addition to neurological repair.
6. Use specialized natural-healing remedies (herbs, homeopathy, essential oils, and so forth) to promote the repair of the immune system and the healing of specific neurological or body functions.
7. Get ample exercise, rest, and sunshine.
8. Engage in specific neurodevelopmental activities that promote the strengthening and organization of weak neurological systems. (Discussed in Chapter 5 and at the end of this chapter.)
9. And learn more in-depth information on the topics discussed in this book, in addition to any additional alternative health-related information that sparks your interest.

The Natural Living Lifestyle

The above is a summary—and not a comprehensive list—of the many principles advocated by those who are healthy and live the natural living lifestyle. In short, the natural living lifestyle is about you *personally taking action* to ensure that you and your family enjoy vibrant health—while refusing to let the government, medical doctors, insurance companies, advertising blitzes, pharmaceutical empires, and others tell you how to manage a disease. *You* must figure out *your* best health practices, on your own, through your research efforts. Discernment and discretion is required. Of course the information in this book is designed to help you on that course, but it is always up to you to truly understand the needs of your body and your family for vibrant health.

My book *The Beginner's Guide to Natural Living* gives a complete overview of the lifestyle as accepted by those who practice, preach, and live it. The natural living lifestyle, as discussed in *The Beginner's Guide*, is presented here in condensed form for your understanding. Also included in this chapter is specific information that relates to neurological repair.

Drink Pure Water

As mentioned in Chapter 6, the fluoride added to our water supply can cause numerous health problems. Add to that any number of biological pathogens, toxic chemicals, and heavy metal particles often found in municipal water, and it's obvious that the water from your tap shouldn't be trusted. Providing yourself and family with properly filtered water is important. The best options include drinking filtered water, such as store-purchased bottled water; water bottles filled at filter stations found in supermarkets; or the use of an in-home, high-quality water filter that will remove all contaminants, including fluoride. Drinking water that's free of fluoride is very important—fluoride can be poisonous to our health. Custom Pure manufactures high-quality water filters that can remove fluoride. (Their products can be found at www.custompure.com.)

Stop Eating Toxic Food

As discussed in Chapter 6, our food supply has been genetically modified, irradiated, and stripped of vital nutrition through processing. Most of what we eat is polluted with a variety of toxic chemicals, synthetic preservatives and dyes, and heavy metals. Daily intake of nutritionally stripped, devitalized, slightly toxic food on a daily basis *will* cause health problems, sooner or later. Because it's nearly impossible to avoid this type of food when we go out to eat, it's very important to *not* eat it at home. Make your kitchen a sanctuary of highly nutritious, alive, whole, organic food.

Two types of substandard foods often overlooked are dairy and sugar. Sugar robs the body of minerals and destroys the immune system. Sugar-coated cereals in the morning and soda pop in the afternoon combined with pastries and other processed food in the evening *literally poisons a child*. As mentioned in Chapter 6, dairy is not assimilated well by most people and in fact is an allergen to many, if not most, children. Cow dairy is for cows—*not* humans. Remove these two substances from your child's diet and watch his or her health improve in no time.

Eat Organic Food

You'll want to stock as much organically grown food in your home as possible—it is the least toxic, best-tasting, most nutrient-dense food available.

Organic farming works in harmony with nature instead of against it. It maintains and replenishes soil fertility and avoids genetic engineering and irradiation. Organic food is free of toxic and persistent pesticides and herbicides, and it is produced without sewage sludge fertilizers (which often contain extremely toxic "recycled" heavy metals and other pollutants, such as industrial waste). In addition, organics have no synthetic preservatives and additives. If an organic product is used in prepackaged food, it is usually minimally processed to maintain its integrity.

Because it's easy to be lulled into buying the numerous prepackaged organic delights available, keep in mind that eating *freshly prepared*, whole food—as nature intended—is best. Most of the food you and your family eat should come from the produce section.

Shop at Natural Food Stores

If you're serious about buying organic food and living a healthier lifestyle, you'll want to switch from shopping at a conventional grocery store to shopping at a natural food store (also known as a health food store). The reason is simple: natural food stores consciously stock products that are better for you and for the environment, and they refuse to carry most products considered by natural living standards to be unhealthy. With over 8,000 such stores nationwide today, there is sure to be one near you—just look in the Yellow Pages under "Health Food Stores," consult the *GreenPeople* online database (www.greenpeople.org/healthfood.htm), or refer to the book *Healthy Highways: The Road Guide to Healthy Eating* (Ceres Press, 2004) by David and Nikki Goldbeck, which lists over 1,900 natural food stores and health-conscious restaurants. Natural food stores carry not only a wide selection of organic produce, but almost all the other types of products you would find at a conventional store—only these products are healthier for us and the environment.

Although some conventional grocery stores are now carrying organic produce and natural products in limited quantities, you'll pay a higher price for them there than at the natural food store. Furthermore, the owners and management of conventional stores are often driven mainly by profits, while owners of natural food stores are motivated by both profits and a worthwhile philosophy—i.e., we should only use products that are healthy for us and the environment. Every business must make a profit to stay in business, but not necessarily at the expense of our health or the world. The success of large natural food store chains such as Whole Foods and Wild Oats have proven that a business can achieve success while remaining true to this philosophy.

Use Potent Supplements

Most soil is depleted of many important minerals, which means that our food—even organic food—doesn't always have optimum nutritional value. One of the best ways to help overcome this deficiency is to take supplements on a regular basis. When dealing with a health issue, such as an attention disorder or general weakness of the body, supplements can prove extremely useful. Typically, you'll either need to shop at a natural food store to find the supplements recommended in this section or visit a natural doctor who can provide you with specific, high quality supplements (not to be confused with natural healing remedies, discussed later in this chapter). Enumerated below are five types of supplements suggested for regular intake: green super foods, including chlorella and wheatgrass; probiotics; enzymes; essential fatty acids; and amino acids.

Green Super Foods

Most natural food stores sport a "green foods" section, which makes it easy to find this type of supplement. You'll find products such as alfalfa, barley grass, spirulina, and wild blue-green algae, as well as custom blends that contain many or all of these plants and algae. Besides offering a variety of minerals, vitamins, amino acids, and essential fatty acids in a concentrated format, they all contain chlorophyll—a unique and important plant molecule. As Paul Pitchford discusses in his book *Healing with Whole Foods*, chlorophyll provides numerous health benefits. It stops bacterial growth in wounds; eliminates bad breath and body odor; removes drug deposits; and counteracts all toxins, including radiation. It also acts as a blood builder and purifier, renews tissue; promotes healthful intestinal flora; activates enzymes that produce vitamins A, D, and K; reverses anemic conditions; reduces high blood pressure; strengthens the immune system; relieves nervousness; and serves as a mild diuretic.[1]

Your best bet is to consume a mixed green super food, such as Barlean's Greens, until you learn more about the variety of super foods available. Simply mix any of these green powders into water or juice and enjoy.

Two powerful green super foods merit special mention here: chlorella and wheatgrass.

CHLORELLA: Chlorella contains ten to 100 times more chlorophyll than leafy green vegetables. It is grown in a controlled medium where minerals are added to optimize it for human consumption. Its small size requires centrifuge harvesting and special processing to improve the digestibility of the tough outer wall, which makes it more expensive than spirulina. However, chlorella's cell wall binds to heavy metals, pesticides, and carcinogens such as PCBs and escorts the toxins out of the body, making it a particularly valuable supplement. Use as directed.

WHEATGRASS: You can find fresh wheatgrass juice in most natural foods stores and juice bars, or you can juice at home with a special juicer. Grass from grains such as barley, wheat, oat, kamut, and rye—when harvested just before they produce a grain—is a nutritional powerhouse. (Think of how massive cows, antelope, deer, bison, elephants, and many other animals become—just from eating grass!)

In addition to being good for other mammals, grass has all the major and trace minerals humans require. Grass, in general, is packed full of vitamins (including every type of B Vitamin—even B-12), and boasts essential fatty acids, every type of essential amino acid, and more than eighty enzymes. It also provides protein in the form of polypeptides, which are assimilated faster than meat-based protein. Finally, grass is very abundant in chlorophyll, discussed above.

The sugar in wheatgrass helps to quickly deliver chlorophyll into the bloodstream. These sugars crystallize in the intestinal tract, which draws toxins out of the tissues. One ounce of wheatgrass juice can contain up to 18,000 units of betacarotene (a precursor of Vitamin A, an immune builder); it also has abundant Vitamin E (which fights cancer growth) and a large amount of Vitamin K (for proper blood clotting). Wheatgrass juice is also loaded with enzymes that help detoxify harmful substances and participate in thousands of the constant chemical changes taking place in the body.

Although it is a nutritional powerhouse, the most unique aspect of fresh wheatgrass juice is probably its "aliveness." This "liquid sunshine" abounds with an electromagnetic "life force" (sometimes referred to in Eastern philosophies as "prana," "chi," or "qi" energy). When the concentrated energy of wheatgrass enters the body, it has a profound healing affect on everything it contacts. Freshly picked vegetables, especially leafy greens, have this energy as well, but it's so concentrated in fresh wheatgrass juice that you can feel it as soon as you drink it.

For health maintenance, one to two ounces of wheatgrass juice on a regular basis (often taken in "shots") is plenty; four or more ounces a day is recommended *for adults* during cleansing or when overcoming health challenges. A word of warning: Reduce consumption of this powerful detoxification agent if you begin to feel ill due to the detoxification process (too many toxins may be simultaneously flooding your system). Generally, wheatgrass juice is taken on an empty stomach at least half an hour before a meal. You can find it at your local juice bar or natural food store; or for around $200, you can buy a wheatgrass juicer (note that this appliance is different from a vegetable juicer). Venders who offer wheatgrass juice can usually sell you trays of the grass for home juicing.

Probiotics

"Probiotic," derived from the Greek "for life," is a term used to describe the friendly bacteria and fungi that inhabit our large and small intestines. At least 400 different species of microflora live in the human gastrointestinal tract. There are billions of these microbes, amounting to approximately three pounds per adult! Two of the most important of these bacteria are acidophilus (*Lactobacillus acidophilus*), which inhabit the small intestine, and bifidus (*Bifidobacterium bifidum*), which inhabit the large intestine. Proper levels of these important probiotics help to keep pathogenic organisms (e.g., candida) in check.

All of our organs are of course, important, but when you are seeking to improve your overall health, the intestine requires your attention first. If it doesn't function properly, it undermines the ability of all other organs to work optimally. Daily supplementation of acidophilus and bifidus is important because they are easily destroyed by factors such as antibiotics and other prescription drugs, stress, a diet high in meat or fats, and poor diet in general. In fact, if antibiotics have been routinely used, then taking probiotic supplements is highly recommended to help bring the flora back into balance and reverse candida symptoms. Probiotics can be found in the supplements section of health food stores, and the Bio-K brand is a particularly excellent supplement.

Enzymes

Enzymes are considered the "sparks of life." Even with appropriate levels of minerals, vitamins, amino acids, water, and other nutrients, without enzymes, life ceases to exist. For this reason, enzymes are sometimes loftily described as possessing "life force energy." (Appropriately, unlike many vitamin and mineral supplements, enzymes cannot be made from synthetic sources.) These energized protein molecules play a necessary role in virtually all biochemical activities. They are required to digest food and to repair cells, tissues, and organs. In fact, they regulate and govern all living cells in plants and animals, and are responsible for providing the energy for all biochemical reactions that occur in nature. Fruit ripening, seeds sprouting, flowers blooming, and people healing—all are examples of enzymatic activity.

There are three major enzymatic classifications: metabolic, digestive, and those obtained from food. Metabolic and digestive enzymes are produced in the body, but food enzymes are not—*they only come from plant food*. Processing or cooking food above 112 degrees destroys food enzymes. Therefore, to ensure proper digestion of food and metabolic activity, it is helpful to consume enzyme supplements to assist in the proper assimilation of the nutrients required for healing.

Essential Fatty Acids

Flaxseed oil and fish oil are good sources for essential fatty acids, the basic building blocks of fats. Essential fatty acids are needed for normal cell structure and function—yet our bodies don't manufacture them. Two types of essential fatty acids, omega-3 and omega-6, are required for proper functioning of nerve cells and cell membrane walls (the number describes the place of the first double bond in these polyunsaturated fatty acids).

All our cells are enveloped by a membrane composed mostly of essential fatty acid compounds called phospholipids, which play a major role in determining the integrity and fluidity of the membranes. The type of fat we consume determines the type of phospholipid in the cell membrane. Unfortunately, the Standard American Diet (aptly abbreviated as SAD) lacks adequate amounts of essential fatty acids. Instead, it's high in animal fats, which contain elevated levels of saturated fatty acids, cholesterol, and trans-fatty acids. (Trans-fatty acids are also formed by chemical extraction or high-heat processing and hydrogenation of unsaturated plant oils.) The result of this lopsided fat intake: our cells have the wrong ratio of fatty acids. This imbalance leads to cell membranes with less than optimal amounts of fluid, impairing their ability to perform their primary function: acting as a selective barrier that regulates the passage of nutrients and wastes in and out of the cell.

Furthermore, *and very importantly,* essential fatty acids build the myelin sheath around the neurons in the brain—and the thicker the sheath, *the faster the transmission of information.* Therefore, daily supplementation of omega-3 fatty acids is *crucial* for anyone challenged with neurological dysfunction, including an attention disorder. Fish oil derived from cold-water species such as salmon and mackerel is a source of these fatty acids. (It is sold in natural food stores and comes in liquid and pill forms.)

An excellent source for fatty acids is flaxseed oil. Because of its unique flavor, it can be taken directly by the tablespoon full or poured on food after it's been cooked (heat destroys the oil's helpful properties). Flaxseed oil complements many dishes, such as baked potatoes, salads, stir-fry dishes, and burritos. Barlean's Flax Oil (found at natural food stores) is thought by some to be one of the best-tasting flax oils available. Pour it on your food everyday.

Amino Acids

If you were to somehow remove all the water and fat from the body, seventy-five percent of what remained would be amino acids. Amino acids are the building blocks of proteins. Essential amino acids come from our diet or supplementation, and nonessential amino acids are created in the body. However, when the diet is poor (as explained in the previous chapter), then even nonessential amino acids may not be fully available.

Among the many the amino acids that the body uses are alanine, arginine, asparagines, carnitine, cystine, glutamine, glycine, lysine, proline, taurine, and tryptophan. Deficiencies in any of these or other amino acids may contribute to a number of health issues, such as neurological problems (e.g., attention and behavioral disorders), cardiovascular disease, chronic fatigue, depression, headaches, hypertension, insomnia, metal retardation, poor immunity, seizures, and growth failure.

Of all the nutrients we require, amino acids are of particular importance because neurotransmitters—which are the chemical "language" of the brain—are created from amino acids. Neurotransmitters dictate our memory, mood, behavior, cognitive ability, and mental and emotional states. Conventional drugs prescribed for depression and other mood disorders work by exhausting current supplies of neurotransmitters—but

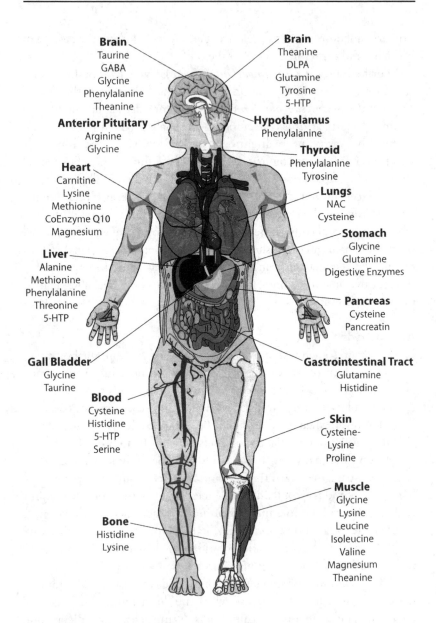

Brain
Taurine
GABA
Glycine
Phenylalanine
Theanine

Brain
Theanine
DLPA
Glutamine
Tyrosine
5-HTP

Anterior Pituitary
Arginine
Glycine

Hypothalamus
Phenylalanine

Thyroid
Phenylalanine
Tyrosine

Heart
Carnitine
Lysine
Methionine
CoEnzyme Q10
Magnesium

Lungs
NAC
Cysteine

Stomach
Glycine
Glutamine
Digestive Enzymes

Liver
Alanine
Methionine
Phenylalanine
Threonine
5-HTP

Pancreas
Cysteine
Pancreatin

Gall Bladder
Glycine
Taurine

Gastrointestinal Tract
Glutamine
Histidine

Blood
Cysteine
Histidine
5-HTP
Serine

Skin
Cysteine-
Lysine
Proline

Muscle
Glycine
Lysine
Leucine
Isoleucine
Valine
Magnesium
Theanine

Bone
Histidine
Lysine

Amino Acids for Brain and Body Functions

Reprinted with permission Pain & Stress Publications (San Antonio, TX) they do not create additional neurotransmitters. To generate more neurotransmitters, and assist the brain in reaching optimum performance, amino acid intake is key. It's important to note that amino acids require the B vitamins, especially B6, as well as magnesium, to be effective.

Billie J. Sahley, PhD, the author of *Heal with Amino Acids and Nutrients* (Pain & Stress Publications, 1991), advises, "Amino acids must be taken daily and in specific amounts for the brain to be chemically balanced." Although taking an over-the-counter amino acid complex supplement—found at natural food stores—is sure to be helpful, to gain insight into your specific amino acid profile, visit a medical doctor who practices natural medicine or a natural doctor (such as a naturopath) to get tested for amino acid deficiency. Once the results are reviewed, the physician will be able to order a custom blended amino acid supplement that can be taken at *therapeutic levels.* Therapeutic levels are much higher dosages to help correct an imbalance, whereas an over-the-counter variety is designed for *maintenance* levels for overall general health. *Testing for amino acid deficiencies and then taking therapeutic levels of custom-blended amino acid supplements is highly recommended for anyone suffering from neurological challenges.*

Detoxification

As you learned in the previous chapter, synthetic toxic chemicals, dangerous heavy metals, artificial growth hormones, and any number of other pathogens easily enter our bodies. The continual intake of these highly toxic substances on a regular basis can overwhelm the body and brain, thereby adversely affecting overall health and neurological functioning. When the body is overloaded with these poisons, the detoxifying organs, such as the liver, kidney, and skin, are compromised. Further, a deficit of amino acids, particularly cysteine—a natural detoxifier that binds to heavy metals so they can be removed from the body—inhibits natural detoxification. When this happens, the immune system is weakened, other systems don't function properly, and disease and/or neurological dysfunction can occur. Therefore, in addition to changing one's diet and removing other sources of toxic intake, it's very important to remove stored toxins from the body and the brain. This process is called detoxification.

Detoxification should be directed toward the body as a whole as well as the brain specifically, particularly with respect to heavy metals. Detoxifying the body will help augment overall health, while detoxifying the brain will assist in improving neurological functioning. According to the studies and parents of Generation Rescue (www.generationrescue.org), autistic symptoms of hundreds of children *disappeared* after they were detoxified of mercury and other heavy metals. Because toxic heavy metals impair neurological function, of course it makes sense to remove them so that neurological function can improve.

There are a number of options available to help the body detoxify, including supplementation with chlorella and wheatgrass juice, colon cleansing, applying castor oil packs, working up a sweat or sitting in a sauna, and eating foods that naturally detoxify. For heavy metal detoxification (especially of the brain), chelation (pronounced key-lay-shun) therapy is frequently used. Although most of these methods of detoxification can be done at home, *if neurological dysfunction is present then it's very important to get tested for heavy metal toxicity to discover exactly which metals must be removed.* Then follow a course of detoxification prescribed by an experienced health care practitioner.

Heavy Metal Testing

The first step to comprehensive detoxification—particularly of heavy metals—is to find a qualified health care professional to run a variety of tests. (A hair analysis test is one of several types of tests available to determine toxic load.) You can choose a naturopathic physician (find one at www.naturopathic.org), or a medical doctor who practices natural medicine. It's very important to spend some time researching several health care practitioners to assess their level of expertise in both testing for toxic load and administering a successful program for detoxification (and in particular, removal of heavy metals)—the removal of heavy metals can cause problems if not done correctly. Once you're satisfied that the practitioner is qualified in testing and detoxification, undergo all recommended tests so that the best understanding of the situation will be available to you both.

If heavy metal toxicity is indicated, your health care practitioner may recommend chelation therapy, discussed in a moment. A naturopathic physician may additionally recommend a number of other treatments, including the use of herbs, dietary changes, and homeopathic remedies, to name a few. You can supplement the detoxification process by using any of the methods listed below. Chelation therapy is discussed last as it's an aggressive medical treatment.

Of particular note is that a person may have heavy metal toxicity, including mercury toxicity, *yet the test may not show it.* This is because the detoxification function has been so impaired in the individual that even the test—which relies on the detox abilities of the body—*will produce a false negative.* For more information on this essential information, please read the analysis by Rashid Buttar, DO, which is reprinted (as abridged version) in Chapter 9.

Apple Cider Vinegar

Pure, organic, unfiltered apple cider vinegar has been used successfully for thousands of years to cleanse and purify the body of toxins. Organic apple cider vinegar contains numerous vitamins, minerals, and trace minerals, especially potassium, which aids in the cleansing and healing process. Potassium is the "mineral of youthfulness," keeping the arteries flexible and resilient. Its primary functions are ensuring the tissues of the body remain healthy, soft, and pliable, and helping to prevent heart attacks and strokes. Our bodies are meant to be self-cleansing, self-correcting, self-repairing, and self-healing. With potassium—the master mineral—toxic poisons are literally placed "in solution" so they can be flushed out of the body.

Numerous books have been written about the wonders of apple cider vinegar. Drinking a couple teaspoons a day, straight or mixed in with juice or water, will be of great benefit. Just be sure to get pure, organic, and unfiltered apple cider vinegar, such as Bragg's Apple Cider (found at natural food stores)—the highly processed varieties do not have these health benefits.

Colon Cleansing

Cleaning the colon is one of the most important things we can do to achieve vibrant health (it is particularly beneficial for adults). Richard Anderson, ND, NMD, in his book *Cleanse and Purify Thyself* (Christobe Publishing, 2000), notes that the colon will become clogged after years of poor dietary choices; because of this buildup, disease will almost invariably manifest.

According to Anderson, when we eat poorly on a continual basis (or the wrong foods on an occasional basis), the intestines react by secreting a protective mucoid layer to prevent the absorption of toxins. This protective mechanism was designed for the occasional ingestion of bad or rotten food, not for the daily abuse that the Standard American Diet places on our digestive system. When we eat incorrectly on occasion, the pancreatic juices will strip the mucoid layer off within a few days; but a daily barrage of overly processed and chemically laden foods creates a buildup of the stuff (called fecal mucoid matter)—and that causes problems.

After years of eating a poor diet we will accumulate this mucoid matter (which often causes a bulging of the gut in older adults). As a result, food moves more slowly through the intestines, nutrients aren't well absorbed, moisture is decreased, worms and parasites colonize, unfriendly bacteria thrive, free radicals form, toxins can't be properly eliminated, and consequently, various diseases of the intestine may appear. Fecal mucoid matter buildup results in fermentation, putrification (rotting), and stagnant pus pockets filled with various poisons and harmful bacteria (hence the foul smells when gas is passed). Or disease can manifest anywhere in the body. The late Bernard Jensen, PhD, observed that "every tissue of the body is fed by the blood, which is supplied by the bowel. When the bowel is dirty, the blood is dirty, and so on to the organs and tissues. *It is the bowel that invariably has to be cared for before any effective healing can take place*" (italics mine).[2]

If you understand this one concept—*that most degenerative disease originates from a dirty colon (and the wrong diet)*—you'll understand more about the cause of degenerative disease than most of the Western medical community (which advocates drugs to manage such symptoms, and surgery to cut out affected parts).

One major problem with a dirty colon is that it becomes an excellent breeding ground for parasites, worms, and unfriendly bacteria. When the colon is a cesspool of these organisms, they steal our valuable nutrients and live off them. Some worms get lodged into the fecal mucoid matter so deeply that even strong herbs won't kill them.

Disease almost always originates in the colon (excepting toxic overload due to vaccinations or outright chemical contamination). When the colon is overloaded with toxins on a regular basis, those toxins seep into the bloodstream and lymph, eventually settling into weaker areas of the body. The body deliberately stores toxins in fat cells for to keep them away from the rest of the body, but when too much builds up in one area, cancer or other serious diseases can develop. The name of the disease depends upon where the poisons settle: in women, for instance, one of the largest areas of fat is found in breast tissue—which is why breast cancer is so prevalent.

Cleansing your colon isn't that difficult, but it does require some effort. Typically, it involves taking herbs to break up the fecal matter, consuming bentonite clay to absorb toxins, consuming psyllium husk to pull dislodged fecal matter out of the intestines, taking mineral supplements to replace lost minerals, and doing an enema or visiting a colon hydrotherapist to irrigate and remove toxins from the colon. Since colon cleansing is more important for adults than children, it's beyond the scope of this book to give a full breakdown of the process. For exact instructions on how to cleanse the colon, please refer to any of these three excellent sources of information: Chapter 7 of my book *The Beginner's Guide to Natural Living* (available at www.thenaturalguide.com), Richard Anderson's Arise and Shine program (www.ariseandshine.com), or Richard Schulz's "incurables" cleansing program (www.herbdoc.com).

Chelation Therapy

Chelation therapy is the preferred method of removing heavy metals—such as cadmium, lead, mercury, and arsenic—from the body and brain. Chelation therapy uses one or more substances that have the ability to bind to a toxic metal and help escort it out of the body. There are three ways of taking a chelating agent: transdermally (through the skin), orally, and intravenously (though an intravenous drip, or IV).

Although any substance that binds to a toxin and escorts it out of the body can be considered a chelating agent (e.g., chlorella or wheatgrass juice), typically chelation therapy refers to the use of a few substances designed specifically for heavy metal detoxification. The most popular are EDTA, DMSA, and DMPS. EDTA (ethylenediamine tetra-acetic acid)—a synthetic amino acid used since the 1940's to remove lead from children—is a common chelating agent used primarily for eliminating lead, and secondarily for other heavy metals such as cadmium and arsenic. DMSA (meso-2,3-dimercaptosuccinic acid) has been used since the 1950's to remove heavy metals. DMPS (dimercaptopropanesulfonate) is specifically designed to remove mercury. There are conflicting reports as to the effectiveness and safety of DMSA and DMPS; however, both are considered more effective for mercury removal than EDTA.

Oral chelation works more slowly than intravenous or transdermal chelation. However, it's less expensive, and if the cost of the other methods is prohibitive, it's better to begin chelation orally than not to do it at all. That said, the best way to administer chelation therapy is through the skin (transdermally), according to the American Board of Clinical Metal Toxicology's onetime Vice Chairman Rashid Buttar, DO, and the parents of formerly autistic children of Generation Rescue (www.generationrescue.com). Specifically, Buttar and Generation Rescue's members recommend, and have had great success with, the transdermal application of DMPS. For more information on this method of chelation therapy, please visit www.tddmps.com (TD-DMPS stands for transdermal DMPS) and read Chapter 9.

If you or your child has neurological challenges and/or behavioral issues, there is a strong probability that heavy metal poisoning may be part of the cause. If autistic behavior is exhibited, then mercury poisoning should be suspected and chelation therapy is strongly advised. *Of particular note is that mercury may not show up in a heavy metal test—the impaired detoxification mechanism in the body will prevent the mercury from being discharged during the assessment.* This is an extremely important point that cannot be overemphasized, and therefore it would be wise to review the work of Rashid Buttar—reprinted in Chapter 9—if you have any questions about the relationship between impaired detox function and *false negatives* on heavy metal tests (also see www.tddmps.com).

Any type of chelation therapy will require the guidance of an experienced health care professional. For chelation therapy resources, please visit www.generationrescue.com, look online, using a Web search engine (search for "chelation therapy," plus your city), or talk with your doctor.

Exercise

Physical exercise not only strengthens muscles and overall health, but also activates the lymph system, which is partly responsible for detoxification. Additionally, *coordinated movement* helps organize and strengthen neurological systems and pathways. Martial arts or yoga, which incorporate repetitive, coordinated movements, are excellent choices for children suffering from neurological challenges. If their health allows, children can exercise to the point of perspiration—but of course they should never "overdo" it. Speak to a health care provider before your child begins any exercise program.

Visit a Naturopathic Physician for Biological Repair

As mentioned earlier, the central tenet of conventional medicine is that symptoms/ailments must be managed with drugs. Natural medicine, on the other hand, seeks to understand why the symptoms appeared in the first place; the practitioner then works with the patient to correct the cause(s) of those symptoms.

In the case of ADD/ADHD-diagnosed children—and others suffering from neurological challenges—visiting a naturopathic physician can be invaluable. Through detoxification, nutrition therapy, lifestyle changes, and natural remedies, this type of natural doctor will work to ensure that body and brain are operating at optimal levels.

Because you may be unfamiliar with natural physicians' educational background and approach, what follows is an overview of what these doctors do—and why they're qualified to work with ADD/ADHD-diagnosed children.

Naturopathic physicians (NDs) treat "the whole person," taking into account the body-mind-spirit interconnection and the individual needs of the patient. Spending up to ninety minutes for an initial visit and an average of forty-five minutes for follow-up exams, the naturopath asks numerous questions, performs a detailed physical exam, thoroughly investigates symptoms and complaints, explains treatment options, and includes the patient in choosing a treatment plan.

Naturopathic physicians are primary care providers (family physicians) and, like an MD or other conventional doctor, an ND will often use a number of laboratory procedures, as well as a physical exam, to make a diagnosis. Additionally, nutritional status, metabolic function, and toxic load are frequently considered in reaching a diagnosis and treatment decisions.

The naturopathic doctor may "prescribe" noninvasive therapies such as lifestyle or behavior modification and relaxation techniques. Spinal manipulation, massage therapy, therapeutic nutrition, botanical medicine, detoxification, physiotherapy, exercise therapy, homeopathy, acupuncture, and psychological counseling may also be included in treatment. In some states where naturopathic physicians are licensed, naturopaths may also perform minor outpatient surgery and prescribe medication. When prudent, an ND will refer patients to a specialist for a definitive diagnosis and advice.

The first two years of naturopathic school are very similar to conventional medical school, requiring coursework in anatomy, physiology, pathology, biochemistry, neurology, radiology, minor surgery, microbiology, obstetrics, immunology, gynecology, pharmacology, pediatrics, dermatology, clinical laboratory, and physical diagnosis, among other areas of study. The second two years focus on clinical skills: NDs receive training in a wide range of natural therapeutics such as botanical medicine, homeopathy, natural childbirth, acupuncture, physiotherapy, and clinical nutrition.

Because coursework in natural therapeutics is *added* to a standard medical curriculum, naturopathic doctors receive significantly more hours of classroom education in these areas than do graduates of many leading medical schools. Students also complete a clinical internship consisting of 1,500 hours treating patients under the supervision of licensed naturopathic and conventional medical physicians in an outpatient setting. As you can see, credentialed naturopathic physicians are highly educated doctors who have a profound understanding of the body and mind—and what is required for vibrant health.

Although practitioners of traditional Chinese medicine and acupuncture are also options for primary care, one of most important reasons to visit a naturopathic physician is his or her ability to run a variety of toxic load tests and amino acid deficiency tests, among other assessments, to check for toxic load and metabolic function. Once this information is at hand, the naturopath can holistically treat ill health and/or poor neurological function with a customized detoxification plan (which may include chelation therapy), a nutritional supplement plan (which may include amino acid supplementation), lifestyle recommendations (such as the removal of dairy and sugar from the diet), and natural remedies (herbs and homeopathic remedies). Visiting a naturopathic physician, or a medical doctor who practices natural medicine, is highly recommended.

To find a qualified naturopath, visit the American Association of Naturopathic Physician's web site at www.naturopathic.org and choose a naturopath from their database.

Use Natural Healing Remedies

Natural healing remedies offer relatively nontoxic methods for strengthening and building the immune system, bodily systems, and overall neurological functioning.

In recent years, even people who would not consider themselves natural lifestyle advocates have turned to natural healing remedies, particularly herbs. One especially well-known herb is ginkgo biloba, which is known to help brain function because it increases blood flow to the brain. Echinacea, another popular herb, helps "jump start" the immune system. Many manufacturers create blended herbal supplements designed for certain ailments or functional support.

Less widely known among the general public is energetic medicine. Energetic medicine works by stimulating a response in the body's electrodynamic field. It encompasses traditional Chinese medical remedies, such as acupuncture; flower essences, which assist in improving mental and emotional well-being; and homeopathic remedies, which help bodily systems heal. (See this chapter's "Homeopathy" section for more information.)

These natural healing remedies can be found at natural food stores and may be prescribed by natural doctors. Depending upon the ailment, any variety of herbs, homeopathic remedies, and flower essences may be of benefit.

An excellent resource for specific natural remedies is *Prescription for Nutritional Healing* (Avery, 2000), by James F. Balch, MD, and Phyllis A. Balch, available at most natural food stores. Although personnel at natural food stores can't "prescribe" supplements for health conditions, they can tell you which remedies provide functional support for certain bodily systems. Many natural food stores also offer a searchable computer database of remedies for specific ailments. Finally, an excellent resource for information is a natural doctor, such as a naturopathic physician.

Homeopathy[3]

Homeopathy is well-established and respected in Great Britain, France, Switzerland, Germany, India, and many other countries. It is not yet well known in the United States but is gaining popularity because of its high success rate in helping people, especially those who cannot be assisted by conventional medicine. Conventional medicine may deem a particular condition incurable—but that is *not* a factor in determining whether the homeopathic approach can help.

Homeopathy is often an effective treatment for people who have chronic diseases, long-term physical or emotional problems, or recurring illnesses. After taking the correct homeopathic remedy, patients feel greater well-being and even happiness—for homeopathic care goes far deeper than most other treatments.

Homeopathy was developed by German physician and chemist Samuel Hahnemann in the early 1800's. Through numerous experiments, he furthered the theory of "The Law of Similars"—meaning that a substance in small doses can alleviate symptoms similar to those it causes at higher doses. He ascertained that the microdose of a substance would stimulate the body's immune system to heal whatever pattern of symptoms would be found if the body was given a large dose of the same substance. This principle is also known as "likes cure likes"—it is the first cornerstone of homeopathy.

Homeopathic remedies are prepared by a detailed process of repeated dilution and shaking, which makes them capable of stimulating the body's own defense system. The shaking, or "succussion," is the second cornerstone of homeopathy.

Although the molecules of the original substance may be gone, the process of dilution and succussion leave something behind—an imprint of the molecules' energy pattern, their "essence"—that gives the new, post-succession substance a healing charge. Scientists who accept the potential benefits of homeopathy suggest several theories to explain how the highly diluted remedies may act. Using recent developments in quantum physics, they have proposed that electromagnetic energy in the medicines may interact with the body on some level.

Nonetheless, homeopathic medicine works in a way that is not entirely understood or recognized by some in modern allopathic medical science. This is not cause to dismiss it (especially given homeopathy's track record of success). Magnets exerted their force long before science could explain the mechanism. Physicists are still trying to explain gravity and the nature of matter and continue to discover new phenomena that challenge once intractable ways of seeing the world. We are all familiar with energy forms, such as electromagnetic radiation and subatomic particles, that were once invisible and immeasurable—and that, despite scientific advances, continue to elude our full understanding.

Like other natural health practitioners, homeopaths appreciate the body's intelligence and know that it produces symptoms for a reason. In most cases, homeopaths consider everything that is going on in the patient's life rather than merely observing isolated symptoms. The patient complaining of headaches may also suffer from depression, insecurity, low energy, and a long list of other conditions. These issues may stem from the same underlying cause; if so, addressing that cause will enable the patient's varied problems to heal.

During a lengthy initial appointment (usually about ninety minutes) the homeopath will explore the patient's complaints. Then appropriate remedies, made from plants, minerals, and other natural substances, are prescribed. Sometimes a remedy is given in a single dose and allowed to work over a period of time. In other instances, an initial dose is given, followed by repeated doses over a period of hours, days, or weeks. In any case, homeopaths recognize the importance of intervening as little as possible.

Use of homeopathic remedies can never harm the body. Even if they don't seem to work, they will not hurt. An experienced practitioner can help you use them in a way that won't spoil the curative action of the potencies.

See The HANDLE Institute for Neurological Repair

While a naturopathic physician will address toxicity levels and nutritional deficiencies of the brain from a biological perspective, the HANDLE approach uses a noninvasive technique to analyze deficiencies in neurological function, then provides individualized programs designed to gently stimulate repair of compromised neurological functioning. Judith Bluestone, founder and clinical director of The HANDLE Institute, is uniquely qualified for this type of work: she developed her approach from eleven years of academic study, over thirty-five years of professional practice, continuing education, and a lifetime of personal experimentation through which she overcame her own serious neurodevelopmental differences, including ongoing seizures as a child.

Bluestone developed a therapeutic approach—which she later named HANDLE (Holistic Approach to Neurodevelopment and Learning Efficiency)—as an outgrowth of her work with the Educational Psychology

Services of the Health Center in Kiryat Shmonah, Israel, in 1982. She spent eleven years in Israel, where she designed therapeutic activities for at-risk young children in a crime-ridden area, teaching preschool and kindergarten teachers how to integrate the activities into the curriculum. She succeeded, where everyone else had failed, in mainstreaming the children. It was there that she developed many of the insights that were to become the HANDLE approach. In 1989, the projects she designed and supervised received Israel's National Prize for Early Childhood Education. She moved to the United States and in 1994 founded The HANDLE Institute.

In its first two years of operation, The HANDLE Institute yielded a *ninety percent success rate in those families that performed their home-implemented programs*. Its approach has since been adopted by numerous practitioners around the world.

Four key concepts underpin HANDLE's success:

1. A comprehensive holographic understanding of how the numerous neurological systems and the brain function—independently and together, including the hierarchy of interaction between those neurological systems.
2. An artful combination of numerous disciplines, melding Western neuroscientific research with some Eastern healing methodologies—while maintaining a nonjudgmental, client-centered approach in which behaviors are viewed as communication.
3. An ability to observe an individual and through the observation of performance on numerous tasks presented, then come to a relatively accurate conclusion as to which neurological systems are compromised.
4. A neurodevelopmental/educational approach that provides the client family with an effective, individualized, non-drug program consisting of HANDLE's therapeutic Gentle Enhancement activities, which strengthen neurological functioning without producing stress, supplemented by suggestions of ways to improve nutritional status, decrease toxic load, and generally strengthen the cellular basis of the client's neurophysiological status.

In Chapter 5 you learned that the collection of symptoms that constitute ADD/ADHD would be better categorized as Attentional Priority Disorder, given the sensory overload that absorbs a child's attention away from tasks or instructions. Similarly, other labels, such as autism, Tourette's syndrome, Asperger's syndrome, and dyslexia fall under a broader category: compromised neurological systems. The HANDLE approach recognizes that each individual labeled with a medical definition has a unique set of neurological challenges; the goal of HANDLE assessments is to determine which neurological systems are compromised and then provide an individualized treatment plan designed to stimulate repair and organize the affected areas.

One of the cornerstones of HANDLE therapy is the understanding that, given the correct stimulus and the "strength" of that stimulus, the neural pathways and neurological systems—including the brain—will adapt, grow, repattern, and repair. HANDLE philosophy places emphasis on proper vestibular functioning because it is foundational to the functioning of many other neurological systems. It is not without reason that a vast majority of ADD/ADHD-labeled children also had recurrent ear infections, given that ear infections often compromise the vestibular system.

Another unique tenet of the HANDLE philosophy is that weakened neurological systems can be stimulated only so much before that system will overload and shut down. In fact, the common thread among ADD/ADHD/APD children is that they are *sensory-overloaded children*. Yet, when there's an understanding of which neurological systems and subsystems are compromised, then the individual can perform specific, therapeutic activities designed to give those systems what they need to make them grow stronger, without stressing or overloading them. This principle of not stressing the systems is referred to in the HANDLE approach as Gentle Enhancement. It's just like weightlifting: muscles need to be stressed just enough to build muscle, but go too far and the muscle may lock or tear, rather than grow.

The recommended activities are simple to perform, and require virtually no special equipment. Each person's program is specially designed to meet his or her unique needs. There are dozens of activities designed to enhance functioning. Some of the more frequently suggested activities involve:

- Drinking from a "crazy straw" (a straw twisted into loops).
- Playing follow-the-leader with a flashlight.
- Rhythmic ball bouncing.
- Performing certain activities with the eyes closed.
- Catching a ball.
- Systematic face tapping.
- Stepping through a hula hoop "maze."

Don't be fooled into thinking that these activities aren't powerful—for someone with compromised neurological systems, the proper application of these and other exercises will slowly and steadily improve functionality of troubled systems. Thousands of satisfied HANDLE clients can attest to that. Home-based therapy, involving Gentle Enhancement activities, typically requires approximately a half hour per day, preferably interspersed throughout the day. Results are often seen in as little as two weeks, with significant gains noticed in three to six months.

Changing one's diet and lifestyle, detoxifying the body and brain, adding ample nutrition and quality supplements, and numerous other actions will help repair the body and brain. *However, it's also very important to recognize that in order for the brain to function optimally, all of its neurological systems and subsystems must be able to operate effectively and carry out their designated function. This is where HANDLE can help—with lasting results.* You can learn more by going to www.handle.org or calling The HANDLE Institute's headquarters in Seattle at (206) 204-6000.

Additional Alternative Therapies

There are plenty of alternative therapies that can help improve health and/or neurological functioning. Some of the more advanced alternative therapies you may want to consider include traditional Chinese medicine, acupuncture, biofeedback, craniosacral therapy, and already available specially blended supplements for ADD/ADHD-diagnosed children, such as "Calms Forte for Kids" (found at natural food stores). Additional alternative therapies for neurological dysfunction can be found on the "Links" page on the HANDLE Web site (www.handle.org).

Chapter 8
How to Take Action: A Step-by-Step Plan

The key to reversing an attention disorder or any other neurological challenge is by adopting a natural living philosophy and lifestyle. This approach has enabled people to recover from a variety of supposedly "incurable" conditions, including cancer, heart disease, paralysis, and polio—in addition to attention disorders, autism, dyslexia, and other neurological challenges. Healing occurred thanks to the innate wisdom of the body: under the *right circumstances*, it restores itself to health. Conventional medical philosophy and many of those who practice it believe in managing illness with drugs, surgery, and radiation; natural medicine adherents know that, when given the correct conditions, the body and brain will heal. The job of the natural medicine practitioner is to help that process along.

Thus, the first step to recovery is to create a belief system acknowledging that the body will repair itself—and that it's up to you to figure out what your body requires for it to do its job of healing. The preceding chapters have given you a solid understanding about how to start the healing journey. *This chapter's purpose is to make that information more accessible by summarizing and outlining some of the most important steps to take toward healing.* (Additionally, it expands on information given in Chapter 5 regarding Attentional Priority Disorder and how The

HANDLE Institute effectively addresses attention disorders and other neurological challenges.)

If you don't see results after applying the principles outlined here, don't give up. Keep searching for other natural therapies that *promote the healing of root causes* rather than the management of symptoms. Remember, the body and brain will heal under the right circumstances. Have faith, and push forward.

Eliminate Stressors and Distractions

As discussed in Chapter 5, sensory overload is common for children and adults who have an attention disorder—which The HANDLE Institute has characterized as Attentional Priority Disorder (APD). When overload occurs, attention to tasks at hand won't occur efficiently, and frustrated outbursts, meltdowns, or shut downs are likely. Therefore, do what you can to remove or minimize environmental offenders if you want the child to attend to your instructions or rules. Doing so successfully requires your acute empathy and perception: what you can normally "tune out," the APD child may not be able to. Try to remove or reduce any of these following stressors/environmental offenders before requesting a child's attention:

- The sights and sounds of a TV.
- Background music.
- Tight and/or synthetic clothing on the child. (Such tactile sensations can absorb the child's attention.)
- Strong odors, regardless of whether or not they strike you as pleasant.
- Patterns in fabric such as clothing, drapes, furniture, carpets, etc. (Patterns can give way to visual overload.)
- Fluorescent lighting, particularly when flickering.
- Sunlight (when it interferes with vision).
- A blowing fan.
- Audible conversations or others talking.
- Echoes (which may be present in certain rooms).
- Traffic noise.
- Other similar types of tactile, visual, auditory, or olfactory (smell system) distractions.

Allow Certain Behaviors

People with APD may exhibit behaviors that make them look unfocused and inattentive (such as squirming in their seats, avoiding eye contact, or insisting on wearing a visor). In reality, their behavior is an effort to mitigate the effects of stimuli that may not only distract them but also cause them to feel uncomfortable or physically insecure: everyday sights and sounds, a lack of balance, poor muscle tone, and so forth. Before assuming a restless or fidgeting child isn't paying attention to you, allow the behavior to continue while talking with the child, then determine whether he or she has been able to pay attention to what you've said.

Some behavioral situations to allow:

* She's looking away while you're talking to her. (She may be reducing visual input so she can focus on what's being said.)
* He's slouching in his chair. (He may not have adequate muscle tone. Slouching reduces stress on the neurological system responsible for muscle tone, allowing him to feel more comfortable and better able to pay attention.)
* He wants to wear a visor. (He's reducing glare and/or reducing the flicker of fluorescent lights, which may be uncomfortable or painful.)
* She's drumming with a pencil, moving around, or fidgeting. (She's keeping her vestibular system activated so she can process information and pay attention.)

Finally, keep in mind that APD children tend to process information at a slower rate than their peers—so patience is required.

Stop Eating Poison

Most food available to us is genetically modified, irradiated, stripped of vital nutrition, and loaded with synthetic chemicals and heavy metals. In reality, it's pretty much poison doctored up to look and feel like food. Vibrant health and neurological repair requires abundant nutrition, *not* abundant toxins! Therefore:

* Stop eating at fast food restaurants.
* Stop eating conventionally grown food (at least at home).

- Stop all dairy consumption (e.g., milk and cheese).
- Stop eating highly processed foods (such as prepackaged meals, white bread, white rice, pastries, sodas, and other food items that have been mass produced, stripped of fiber and nutrients, loaded with sugar and synthetics, or otherwise rendered unhealthy).
- Stop eating any foods with synthetic additives, such as dyes, preservatives, and flavorings.
- Stop eating sugar-coated breakfasts and other sugar-infused items (juices with added sugar or corn syrup, sodas, excessive sweets, and so forth).
- Stop consuming sources of fluoride, including fluoridated tap water, fluoride tablets, and fluoride toothpaste. Fluoride is a deadly poison that may affect neurological functioning and overall health. (There's a reason for the fluoride warning on toothpaste!)

Eat Organic at Home
Fill your entire pantry and fridge only with organic food. Organic food is the best food available, so why not have it in your home to help ensure health and nutrition? Remember, it's much less expensive at natural food stores than at conventional supermarkets.

Eat Alive and Whole Food
Prepare your meals from scratch, using fresh food from the produce section, whole grains, and as little boxed, frozen, or canned food as possible. Alive, whole, fresh food is very important because it has far more nutritional value than prepackaged meals—canned, boxed, or frozen.

Shop at a Natural Food Store
To make adopting a natural lifestyle easier, shop at a natural food/health food store, where you won't have to sift through unhealthy products. Natural food stores stock consistently nutritious items and nontoxic alternatives to household supplies as well as other products. While there, shop for:

- Organic food.
- Nontoxic cleaning supplies.
- Botanical, chemical-free soaps, shampoos, and body products.

- Chlorine-free diapers and feminine products.
- Fluoride-free toothpaste.

Detoxify the Body and Brain
Toxins impair overall health and neurological functioning—and, unfortunately, they're everywhere: in our water, in our air, in pharmaceutical products, in synthetic fabrics, in household cleaning products, in cosmetics, in foods grown with pesticides and laden with synthetic chemicals, in allergens—and the list goes on. Our toxic world overwhelms our natural defenses and infiltrates our bodies and brains. To improve our health, it's important to remove these toxins from our systems. See a natural health practitioner, and use the tips below:

- Wheat grass juice and chlorella are excellent detoxifying agents.
- Colon cleansing removes stored toxins.
- Chelation therapy is an option for heavy metal removal. Consider transdermal chelation (applied to the skin). Chelation therapy requires supervision from a qualified professional, such as a naturopathic physician or a medical doctor who practices natural medicine.
- Eat vegetables that naturally detoxify the body, such as beets, raw potatoes, asparagus, and parsley. Do not underestimate the power of these whole foods. Eat them (especially raw potato) in small quantities, and be sure to drink plenty of water in conjunction with this or any detox protocol.

Take Potent Supplements
Inadequate nutrition precipitates and exacerbates poor neurological health. The following supplements, discussed throughout this book, can be tremendously useful in improving brain functioning (and overall well-being):

- Probiotics help to augment intestinal flora and are highly recommended, especially for those who have undergone an antibiotic treatment. Bio-K is an excellent brand found at natural food stores.
- Enzymes are helpful for proper digestion, which is required for nutrient absorption.

- Green super foods, such as spirulina, barley grass, and chlorella, help provide whole-food nutrition. Green super food powders and formulas, such as Barlean's Greens, are an excellent option. (Mix the formula into juice, then drink.)
- Consume high amounts of essential fatty acids, such as flaxseed oil or fish oil. Essential fatty acids build myelin in the brain, thereby increasing the speed at which information is processed. Flaxseed oil can be added to salad dressings, smoothies, and meals *after* they've been cooked (try it on baked potatoes, stir fries, and burritos).
- Take an amino acid custom-blended supplement. Amino acids are the building blocks for neurotransmitters, the chemical language of the brain. Request an amino acid test from a naturopathic physician, and ask her to acquire the custom blend for you.

Be Wary of Vaccinations

Because of public outcry and thousands of lawsuits, mercury—the second most lethal substance to humans—has been removed from some childhood vaccines. However, it's still present in flu vaccines and other vaccines. Furthermore, contrary to manipulated statistical data and public relations blitzes, there is no credible evidence that the synthetic immunity from vaccines is any better than natural immunity; in fact, it may be quite the opposite.

One of the best reasons to adopt a natural lifestyle is so that natural immunity will be high, therefore avoiding any need (perceived or otherwise) for vaccinations with toxic ingredients and pathogenic viruses and bacteria. One of the best books on the topic is *Immunization: The Reality Behind the Myth* (Greenwood Press, 1995) by Walene James. It offers an accessible, well-researched, highly illuminating overview of this controversial issue.

Visit a Naturopathic Physician

Visit a naturopathic physician or a medical doctor who practices natural medicine. Run all available tests for heavy metal toxicity and amino acid deficiencies. Consider other tests, such as stool tests (which check for candida) and blood tests (which check for mineral imbalances). Your physician should be able to provide you with a detoxification program that includes chelation therapy. You may want to request transdermal

DMPS chelation, and ask the physician to read the Appendix of this book. To find a qualified naturopath, visit the American Association of Naturopathic Physician's Web site at www.naturopathic.org and chose a naturopath from their database.

Visit a Holistic Dentist

Holistic dentists don't use mercury amalgam. Because other dental materials are much safer, why not help ensure that toxic mercury vapor won't accumulate in the tissues of your child?

Try an Energetic Foot Bath

Salt baths have been used since ancient times to draw toxins out of the body due to osmosis. When salt (NaCl) is added to water, the sodium (Na+) and chloride (Cl-) molecules separate and make the water a denser solution than the water inside the body. Water naturally tends to flow through the dermis (skin) from the less dense solution to the denser solution, carrying with it any suspended toxins and foreign material.

In recent years a new technology has developed based on the same philosophy: energized footbaths. The better-designed machines are effective in cellular cleansing because of two separate yet complementary processes that occur simultaneously during a footbath—osmosis and negative ion generation.

When the module is submerged in the footbath water, it charges the solution and promotes the movement of ions in the solution. This ion movement penetrates the dermis and travels to where certain toxins accumulate in the plasma membrane that surrounds each cell body. This increases the metabolic energy of the membrane, so that its function of being selectively permeable is restored to proper working order. The introduction of negative ions from the bath solution also tends to reduce the positive charge that holds the foreign material to the cell, thereby allowing this matter to be released and then gravitate towards the more positively charged bath solution.

The result? Toxins move through the feet and into the water: detoxification. Many practitioners and spas now offer energetic footbaths, and units can also be purchased direct from manufacturers. One highly regarded footbath product is produced by Health & Energy Alternatives and is called the FOCUS™ Energetic System, found at www.healternatives.com.

Visit a HANDLE Practitioner

The HANDLE Institute's approach has a unique understanding of neurological function. HANDLE's evaluation process leads to a neurodevelopmental profile that offers a significant understanding as to which neurological systems are compromised, weak, or not connecting with other systems. The institute's practitioners work with people of all ages (on an out-patient basis) who have neurological challenges, including dyslexia, autism, Tourette's syndrome, traumatic brain injury, learning disabilities, behavioral issues, and attention disorders, as well as those who experience challenges in daily life who have not been given a diagnosis or label. Once a child's unique neurological profile is understood, a customized program is provided to strengthen and reorganize weak systems, utilizing a Gentle Enhancement® program of low- or no-impact exercises. Activities require about a half hour per day and can be carried out at home. Minor changes are often noticed in two weeks while significant improvement can be seen in three to six months. Probably the greatest benefit of the HANDLE approach is that the gains achieved from the program are lasting, even after treatment has stopped. Visit www.handle.org or call (206) 204-6000. HANDLE is very highly recommended for parents who want to see significant gains in their child.

Adopt a Natural Living Lifestyle

How you choose to live becomes an extension of how your child lives. To the degree that you adopt natural living so will your child, and that will play a major role in determining his or her physical and neurological health. This entire book is an explanation of why and how to live a natural lifestyle (even natural medicine falls under the umbrella of natural living). Much of the plan for neurological healing, and recovering from attention disorders, is *natural living in action*. For a more comprehensive understanding of how to live the natural lifestyle and why, read my book, *The Beginner's Guide to Natural Living* (available at natural food stores and www.TheNaturalGuide.com). Meanwhile, you can make the changes described above, and throughout this book, to improve your child's neurological functioning and overall well-being.

Chapter 9
Autism: The Misdiagnosis of Our Future Generations*

Presented to the
US Congressional Sub-Committee Hearing on May 6, 2004
by
Rashid A. Buttar, DO, FAAPM, FACAM, FAAIM
Vice Chairman, American Board of Clinical Metal Toxicology
Visiting Scientist, North Carolina State University

The incidence of Autism has increased from approximately 1 in 10,000 in 1990 to 1 in 166, representing over a 5,700% increase in just the last 15 or so years. In some states, the incidence is now 1 in 80 and **we now have over 1.5 million children diagnosed with Autism in the United States**.

A lot of attention has been given regarding the link between mercury and autism, with mercury being the possible factor underlying the etiology of this condition. The issue of whether mercury plays a role in Autism or other neurodevelopmental disorders has been the subject of long debate and extreme political discourse but the evidence is overwhelmingly obvious to even the simplest of intellects, once the data is objectively reviewed.

*Abridged from original report. See www.drbuttar.com for complete text and additional commentary. Reprinted with permission.

The prevalence of mercury in our society is endemic in nature. The association of mercury with chronic disease in the US "medical literature" exists but is very anemic. However, when searching under Toxline under the Agency for Toxic Substances and Disease Registry (ATSDR), a division of Centers for Disease Control (CDC), one finds all the scientific literature that also includes didactic literature, NOT just the "medical literature." Not surprisingly to advanced researchers and physicians, the association of mercury to chronic diseases is well documented in the didactic scientific literature.

The search for the association between mercury and cardiovascular disease—the number one killer in the industrialized world—revealed 358 scientific papers exemplifying the relationship. The search for the association between mercury and cancer—the number two killer in the industrialized world at the time of this writing—revealed 643 scientific papers exemplifying the relationship. Both of these conditions represent 80% cause of all deaths in the industrialized world, according to the WHO (World Health Organization) as published in 1998. But the association of mercury with neurodegenerative diseases is the most significant, with the references numbering 1445.

The inevitable question is: "How do we get exposed to mercury?" The sources surround us, from mercury amalgams in our teeth, to the contamination of our water sources, inhalation of combustion from fossil fuel, fish that we consume, contaminated water supplies, virtually all vaccinations, and via breast milk, just to name a few. So if mercury is so devastating, why is it allowed to be in our flu shots, vaccines, foods, etc.? This is the "million dollar" question, although it is quite evident to the well informed that the answer will be found somewhere along the money trail.

Increased exposure to mercury through thimerosal containing vaccines is one of the most important issues at hand. Thimerosal (also known as Marthiolate sodium, Mercurothiolate, Thiomersalate and a host of other names) is the common name of a substance known as ethyl mercurithiosalicylic acid. The overburdening knowledge that thimerosal is converted to ethyl mercury (a substance reportedly hundreds, if not a thousand times more destructive than inorganic mercury) in less than one minute after being introduced into the body should give great concern to parents and those appointed to protect the public. Yet, it is virtually ignored.

However, the vaccine issue must not overshadow the cumulative mercury exposure experienced by the patient during gestation and early infancy. These additional exposures besides the vaccine history include but are certainly not limited to: dietary mercury content, dental amalgam fillings which contribute greatly to the maternal mercury load, Rhogam (immunoglobulin) administration to mother during gestation, inoculations for tetanus toxoid, exposure to combustion of fossil fuels, water contamination, and mercuric compounds used in skin products.

Mercury causes damage by various mechanisms, including: competitive and noncompetitive inhibition of enzyme activity by reversibly or irreversibly binding to active sulfur—binding at the sites off and displacing other divalent cations—like magnesium, zinc, copper, and manganese causing a disruption of enzyme systems, disrupting critical electron transfer reactions, and complexing molecules and inducing a change in structure or conformation which causes them to be perceived as foreign by the body's immune defense and repair system (hapten reactions) resulting in hypersensitivity that can potentiate or exacerbate autoimmune reactions. Mercury alters biological systems because of its affinity for sulfhydryl groups which are functional parts of most enzymes and hormones. Tissues with the highest concentrations of sulfhydryl groups include the brain, nerve tissue, spinal ganglia, anterior pituitary, adrenal medulla, liver, kidney, spleen, lungs heart and intestinal lymph glands. But most relevant to us for the purposes of this hearing is that mercury has been clearly shown to causes a denudation of the neurofibrils resulting in direct and devastating damage to the neuronal cells.

Children diagnosed with Autism suffer from acute mercury toxicity secondary to huge exposure while in utero (maternal amalgam load, dietary factors, maternal inoculations, Rhogam injections, etc.) and early on in life (vaccinations preserved with thimerosal, etc.). Adults diagnosed with Alzheimer's suffer from chronic, insidious mercury toxicity secondary to exposure over a long time (amalgam load, inhalation of mercury vapors, combustion of fossil fuels, dietary factors, etc.).

Children with Autism (mercury toxicity) have many resulting imbalances in their systems, including but not limited to, significant allergies, opportunistic infections such as systemic candidiasis, hormonal imbalances, gastrointestinal dysbiosis, immune dysfunctions such as immunosuppression or significant allergies, nutritional deficiencies, etc. However these are what I refer to as the "fires" of autism. All these and other "fires" of autism result from one major "spark." Mercury! Successfully addressing these "fires" will accomplish transient improvement but until the "spark" (mercury) that constantly re-ignites these "fires" has definitively been eliminated, any improvement will be short lived at best. Mercury is NOT the fire. It is however, the spark that ignites and constantly re-ignites these "fires." The fire will keep re-igniting unless the "spark" is eliminated. Thus, mercury is the underlying common denominator and exacerbates the destructive nature of other embedded heavy metals and compounds, contributing in various ways to all the problems from which these children suffer.

The reason some individuals have severe damage from mercury where others do not have serious adverse neurological deficits extends due to various factors which include biological individuality and genetic predisposition. In addition, factors such as the type of toxicity exposure makes an enormous difference. Was it inhaled, ingested, injected or exposed on their skin? What type of mercury exposure did the individual receive? Was it organic or inorganic mercury? If it was organic, was it ethyl mercury or methyl mercury? How frequent was the exposure to the source of toxicity? Was there a significant maternal load present prior to birth? Was the situation exacerbated by the mother being inoculated, or having Rhogam administration either during gestation or even, prior to conception? How many vaccine administrations took place and over what period of time? What about the diet? How about the proximity to industrial sites, and exposure to combustion of fossil fuel? As you can see, the variables are extensive.

Let us answer the question why some people are affected while others show no manifestations of mercury toxicity, despite living in the same environments. In our case, the discussion will be limited to mercury, which is considered to be the second most toxic metal known to man but this explanation is applicable to most other heavy metals as well. Most individuals exposed to mercury as well as other heavy metals have the ability to at least begin the process of eliminating these heavy metals out of their system. **But not everyone has this ability and the extent of variability in the ability of an individual to detoxify their systems will determine the severity of the symptoms of toxicity.** Slides #10 to #14 show the typical individual who can get rid of mercury with appropriate treatments. Despite having been exposed to severe levels of mercury vapor, this patient named Robin T. was able to detoxify once appropriately treated with DMPS, a synthetic amino acid chelation agent. Her mercury level was almost 22 fold greater or 2200% more than what is considered to be safe but with appropriate treatments, her levels returned to normal and her symptoms of mercury toxicity resolved in a relatively short period of time.

However, patients with impaired detoxification pathways do not show similar results on testing. **Their bodies are unable to release the mercury and/or other metals and on testing, the mercury does not appear.** The basis of our treatment protocol for children diagnosed with autism was determined by my clinical observation that certain individuals were unable to detoxify mercury like the vast majority of people appear to have the ability to do so. Slides #16 to # 21 show the case of Karen D. who showed no appreciable levels of mercury despite appropriately being "challenged" with DMPS by two different physicians over a year apart. In Karen D.'s case, she could not detoxify her system effectively despite being treated appropriately with the correct diagnostic methods.

Karen D. was 34 years old when she presented to me with multiple complaints including pain, galactorrhea (milk coming out of her breast), ataxia (abnormal gait while walking), dysphagia (painful swallowing), inability to articulate with a new onset of stuttering, arrhythmia, chest pain, myalgias (muscle aches), arthralgias (joint pain), hirsutism (facial hair), cephalgia (headache), insomnia (inability to sleep), fatigue, malaise (general feeling of sickness), depression, anxiety and suicidal ideations due to being unable to "live like this anymore." On presentation, the patient had notified me she had seen 16 other physicians in the previous 5 years and if I could NOT help her, she would "take care" of the problems herself because she could no longer live this way. **The level of mercury measured during each of Karen D.'s tests was inversely proportionate to the amount of mercury remaining in her system.** It is important to note that this patient received treatments every week but the test results were obtained only every 20 weeks. Despite this disparity between treatments and testing, we see a dramatic and steady increase in mercury levels on testing, directly correlated with significant clinical improvements and alleviations of symptoms.

Karen D. needed to have persistent treatment for a period of almost 2 years, as seen on slides #16 to #21. However, as you will notice, Karen's mercury levels continued to exponentially RISE until her last test which shows the results dramatically drop. What is most interesting is that as the test results revealed a consistently **increasing** level of mercury while the patient began to dramatically improve on a clinical basis. The reason the levels of mercury actually rose in each subsequent test, is that this testing method only determines how MUCH mercury and/or other metals we are able to remove. As treatment continued, we were effectively able to remove a greater quantity of mercury during each and every treatment.

We started treating children with Autism first in 1996. By 1997, we were being referred patients by a pediatric neurologist, who was following a mutual patient and observed significant changes in the child's behavior after implementation of our treatments. However, by the end of 1998, taking care of children with special needs proved more than I wished to handle. Although we had far better success than the traditional approach, our treatments had not been responsible for "normalizing" any children or returning them to a "neurotypic" state. The emotional component was also overwhelming, just having to deal with the pain and frustration of the parents of these children. As a result, we stopped accepting new patients with the diagnosis of Autism or any type of developmental delay before the start of 1999.

On January 25, 1999, my son Abid Azam Ali Buttar was born. By the time he was 14 or 15 months old, he was already saying "Abu" which means father in Arabic, and a few other words such as "bye bye." But by the age of 18 months, my son had not only failed to progress in his ability to speak, but had also lost the few words he had been saying. As he grew older, I began to worry more and more that he was suffering from a developmental delay. He exhibited the same characteristics that so many parents with children that have developmental delays we have observed, such as stemming, walking on tip toes, and lack of eye contact. Sometimes I would call to him but his lack of response would convince me there must be something wrong with his hearing. Certain sounds would make him cringe and he would put his hands on his ears to block the obvious discomfort he was experiencing. He would spend hours watching the oscillation of a fan. But through all this, when he would make eye contact with me, his eyes would say, "I know you can do it Dad." The expression he would give me, for just an instant, would be that of a father encouraging his son.

The oceans of tears that I cried and the hours that I spent trying to determine what was happening to my son are no different than that of any other parent in the same situation. The only difference was that I was one of only 190 some doctors throughout the US as board certified in clinical metal toxicology. And if this was metal related—as was a theory that I had read—I should know how to fix this problem. I tested him and re-tested him and tested him again, searching for mercury. My son's tests showed no appreciable levels of mercury. But the older he became, the more obvious it became that my son was not developing as he was meant to be developing. My son was not meant to be this way and that was the only one thing that I knew for certain. From the time Abie lost his speech which was around 18 months or so, until 36 months of age, he had absolutely no verbal communication except for the one syllable that he would utter, "deh," on a repetitive basis.

About the same time while desperately searching for the cause of the same ailment that had afflicted so many of my own patients previously, I had been invited to present a lecture regarding some of our research on IGF-1 and the correlation with cancer. I had notified the conference that I was too busy to present this lecture but when I learned that Dr. Boyd Haley was also scheduled to present at this conference, I changed my schedule and agreed to lecture just so I could meet and discuss my son's situation with Dr. Haley. That meeting turned out to be one of the key elements which resulted in our development and subsequent current protocol for treating children with autism, autism like spectrum and pervasive developmental delay. My son was the first one who went through this protocol once safety had been established. Dr. Haley told me of a study that had not yet been published at the time.

Just before the year 2,000, Holmes, Blaxill and Haley did a study assessing the level of mercury measured in the hair of 45 normally developing children versus 94 children with neurodevelopmental delays diagnosed as Autism using DSM IV criteria. The finding showed that the Autistic children had 0.47 parts per million of mercury in their hair where as the normally developing children had 3.63 parts per million, more that 7 times the same level of mercury as the Autistic children. Opponents of the mercury-neurodegeneration camp used this opportunity to state that this study clearly showed that mercury had NOTHING to do with Autism or any other neurodegenerative condition. **However, they completely missed the point of the study—the autistic children had impaired detoxification systems!**

These findings were published in the *International Journal of Toxicology* in 2003. Understanding these findings, along with my clinical experience with the case of Karen D. as previously detailed, led me to the conclusion that a more aggressive method of treatment was necessary compared to the DMSA and various other treatments I had to date employed in the attempt to document high levels of mercury in my son, which up to this point, had not been successful. The first two attempts with DMPS as a challenge treatment were unsuccessful, the first due to difficulty catching the urine since Abie was only 2 years old at the time, and the other due to loss of the urine specimen while being delivered to the laboratory. The third try with DMPS, which represented the 6th test we did on my son with all previous tests showing no appreciable levels of mercury, resulted in the findings that his mercury level was over 400% that of safe levels. It is important to note that this level was only indicative of what we were able to "elicit or sequester" out of him. His actual levels were far greater.

I started Abie's treatments on his 3rd birthday, using a rudimentary version of the current TD-DMPS (DMPS in a transdermal base) that my partner, Dr. Dean Viktora and I had played around with a few years previously. By the age of 41 months—5 months after initiating treatment with the TD-DMPS—my son started to speak, with such rapid progression that his speech therapist was noted to comment how she had never seen such rapid progress in speech in a child before. Today at the age of 5, Abie is far ahead of his peers, learning prayers in a second language, doing large mathematical calculations in his head, playing chess and already reading simple 3 and 4 letter words. His attention span and focus was sufficiently advanced to the point of being accepted as the youngest child into martial arts academy when he was only 4. His vocabulary is as extensive as any 10 year old's, and his sense of humor, power to reason and ability to understand detailed and complex concepts constantly amazes me. This was the preliminary basis for the initiation of our retrospective study which came about as a result of the extraordinary results obtained in the treatment of my son Abie, and the subsequent treatment of 31 other children treated in the same manner.

The retrospective Autism study consisted of 31 patients with the diagnoses of autism, autism like spectrum, and pervasive developmental delay. Inclusion criteria was simple, including an independent diagnosis of the above mentioned conditions from either a neurologist or pediatrician, and the desire of the parent to try the treatment protocol using TD-DMPS. All patients reviewed had been sequentially treated as they presented to the clinic and only those patients whose parents who did not wish to be treated with the TD-DMPS were not included. As a side note, of all the parents presented with this option of treatment with DMPS, only one did not wish their child to be treated with DMPS. Some of the older children (over the age of 8) were treated with IV administration of DMPS and their data was obviously not included in this retrospective analysis. However, it's important to note how willing parents were to get their children better.

All 31 patients were tested for metal toxicity using four different tests: urine metal toxicity and essential minerals, hair metal toxicity and essential minerals, RBC metal toxicity, and fecal metal toxicity, all obtained from Doctor's Data Laboratory. These tests were performed at baseline, and repeated at 2 months, 4 months, 6 months, 8 months, 10 months, 12 months, and then every 4 months there after. In addition, all study patients had chemistries, CBC with differentials, lipid panels, iron, thyroid profiles and TSH drawn every 60 days. Further specialized testing also included organic acid testing (OAT test) from Great Plains Laboratory and complete diagnostic stool analysis (CDSA) from Doctor's Data Laboratory. If indicated, IgG mediated food allergy testing was also obtained but was not routinely performed. All 31 patients showed little or no level of mercury on the initial baseline test results.

Compared to the baseline results, all 31 patients showed significantly higher levels of mercury as treatment continued. After two months of treatment with the TD-DMPS, one patient had approximately a 350% increase from previous baseline levels. The improvements in the patients in the study correlated with increased yield in measured mercury levels upon subsequent testing. **Essentially, what was noted was that as more mercury was eliminated, the more noticeable the clinical improvements and the more dramatic the change in the patient.**

The manifestations of this evidence for clinical improvements included many observations but were specifically quantifiable with some patients who had no prior history of speech starting to speak at the age of 6 or 7, sometimes in full sentences. Patients also exhibited substantially improved behavior, reduction and eventual cessation of all stemming behavior, return of full eye contact, and rapid potty training, sometimes in children that were 5 or 6 but had never been successfully potty trained. Additional findings reported by parents included improvement and increase in rate of physical growth, as well as the children beginning to follow instructions, becoming affectionate and social with siblings or other children, seeking interaction with others, appropriate in response, and a rapid acceleration of verbal skills. The results of many of these children has been documented on video, and other physicians involved with this protocol have been successfully able to reproduce the same results.

DMPS, or dimercaptopropane – 1 sulfonate, is a primary chelator for mercury and arsenic. DMPS has pitfalls as well as advantages. The pitfalls include oral dosing—which is the usual recommended dosing—because it is approximately 50% to 55% absorbed by the gastrointestinal mucosa. As a result of already compromised gastrointestinal function and dysbiosis noted in most of these children, DMPS by mouth becomes impractical. Most of the children that have taken the DMPS orally for more than 1 week continuously begin complaining of abdominal pain, cramping and other GI distress. We tried the oral DMPS for almost 6 weeks before eliminating it as a possible therapeutic method. Intravenous methods of application were not an option in children so young, although is the preferred method I have used in my clinical practice for my adult patients with mercury toxicity.

All study patients were also monitored for renal function, and mineral depletion. The key to success with these children was the constant and continuous "pull" of mercury by being able to dose it every other day. Each patient was put on a protocol consisting of the transdermal (on the skin) DMPS (TD-DMPS). Transdermal DMPS is DMPS conjugated with a number of amino acids, delivered in highly specialized micro-encapsulated liposomal phospholipid transdermal base with essential fatty acids. The frequent dosing is one of the most important components of the TD-DMPS. It is important to note that DMPS is highly oxygen reactive and is very unstable when exposed to air. This and many other issues of delivery, stabilization, and oxidation have all been successfully identified and resolved over the last two years with the final result now a pending patent. In addition, certain other components have been added to the TD-DMPS to potentiate the efficacy of treatment, such as the addition of various amino acids and glutathione.

There are a number of agents that have been demonstrated to have clinical utility in facilitating the removal of mercury from someone who has demonstrated clinical signs and symptoms of mercury toxicity. The most important part of this systemic elimination process, however, is the removal of the source of mercury. Once this has been completed, treatment for systemic mercury detoxification can begin.

In our clinical experience, the most effective method that has resulted in the consistent, slow and safest method of removal of mercury in the pediatric population is the TD-DMPS that was originally formulated for the purposes of treating my son's developmental delay. Since its implementation, we have now successfully treated scores of patients, many of whom have completely recovered and all of whom have improved since the implementation of this treatment. These results have been duplicated by other physicians involved with the care of patients with neurodegenerative disease processes.

Summary

The underlying common denominator in chronic neurodegenerative disease seems to be either decreasing vascular supply (less blood to the brain) or accumulation of heavy metals, particularly mercury. The inability of an individual to eliminate toxic metals, especially mercury, is directly related to the level of neurodegeneration experienced. In the young patient population suffering from autism or pervasive developmental delay, the vascular supply is not an issue. The underlying pathology of children with autism and the geriatric population with Alzheimer's is of the same etiology, specifically mercury toxicity.

Both these patient populations suffer from the inability to excrete mercury as a result of a genetic predisposition resulting from various factors. This allele appears to be associated with the inability to get rid of mercury from the system. If these patient populations inhabited a complete mercury free environment, they would not have the problems associated with autism or Alzheimer's. When the mercury is successfully removed from their systems, these individuals begin to significantly improve due to a cessation of the destruction and denudation of the neuro-fibrils, as evidenced by steady improvement in cognitive function.

Mercury is the "spark" that causes the "fires" of autism as well as many other neurodegenerative diseases including PDD, ADD, ADHD and Alzheimer's. Autism is the result of high mercury exposure early in life versus Alzheimer's where there is a chronic accumulation of mercury over a life-time. A doctor can treat ALL the "fires" but until the "spark" is removed, there is minimal hope of complete recovery with most realized improvements being transient at best. Mercury is the underlying common denominator of all the problems from which these children suffer due to impairment of their excretory pathways. And the only solution for these non-eliminators is to effectively remove the mercury while repairing and enhancing the damaged elimination and detoxification pathways. Concomitantly addressing the GI tract is vital if the goal of treatment is to achieve permanent recovery.

Once the process of mercury removal has been effectively initiated, the source of damage is now curtailed and full recovery becomes possible. Complete recovery can now be attained and further enhanced by utilizing various additional essential therapies including nutrition, hyperbarics, etc. **It is my hope and prayer—along with the hopes and prayers of all clinicians who are cognizant of these facts—that the US Congress will act quickly and decisively to put an end to this legalized and tolerated mass modern genocide by outlawing the use of any form of mercury in any capacity in humans, including mercury based preservatives in all childhood and adult vaccines as well as dental amalgams, while also limiting the amount of mercury being released into our environment in order to prevent human exposure so as to reduce the total body burden.**

Rashid A. Buttar, DO, FAAPM, FACAM, FAAIM
Center for Advanced Medicine and Clinical Research
20721 Torrence Chapel Road, Suite # 101 – 103
Cornelius, NC 28031
Clinic Phone: (704) 895-9355
www.drbuttar.com

Resources

TESTS

Your pediatrician or other doctors may not be familiar with these tests. The laboratory personnel can consult with your doctor or can provide names of doctors closest to your area that have knowledge of these tests and therefore provide proper guidance in treating your child. Most of the tests listed are covered by insurance.

Food and inhalant allergy testing: Children with ADHD and autism often have food allergies, and symptoms worsen after the children eat certain foods. Candida (yeast overgrowth) contributes to food allergies.

Amino acid deficiencies: The basic building blocks of protein form neurotransmitters in the brain that regulate mood and behavior.

Candida: (leaky gut) overgrowth of yeast: Organic acid test can detect yeast overgrowth and inborn errors of metabolism. Many ADHD and autistic children have tested positive for abnormally high levels of yeast.

Digestive function: Autistic and ADHD people often exhibit chronic digestive problems. The Organic Acid Test or Comprehensive Stool Analysis can provide information that leads to treatment for bowel disorders. Poor digestion can be a result from an overuse of antibiotics.

Essential fatty acids: Deficiencies in essential fatty acids are very common among ADHD kids.

Heavy metal analysis: ADHD/ADD people improve when toxic metals are removed from the body.

Pesticide and flame-retardant chemicals: All individuals who have symptoms of ADHD, autism, other learning disabilities, convulsions, any chronic pain, and poor coordination should be checked for toxic chemical exposure.

Seizures: Children diagnosed with ADHD may have underlying seizures. Higher than usual incidence of seizures is seen in autism and Tourette's syndrome. Organic acid testing, amino acids testing, essential fatty acid testing, food allergy tests, and metals testing are also important in assessing causes and potential treatment for seizures.

Zinc testing and nutritional testing: Zinc and nutritional deficiencies are common in people with ADHD/ADD.

LABORATORIES
Accu-chem Laboratories
E.H.S. Inc.
990 Bowser Ste. 800
Richardson, TX 75081
(800) 451-0116
www.accuchem.com/testpanel.html
Chlordane (includes related pesticide compounds); organophosphorus pesticide metabolites, heavy metals analysis; chlorinated (organ chlorine) pesticides.

Doctor's Data, Inc.
P.O. Box 111
West Chicago, IL 60185
(800) 323- 2784
www.doctorsdata.com
Hair toxic elemental exposure profile; urine toxic and essential elements; Urine and plasma amino acid analysis; yeast culture and sensitivities; comprehensive drinking water analysis.

Environmental Health Center
8345 Walnut Hill Ln., Ste. 200
Dallas, TX 75231
(214) 368-4132
www.ehcd.com
Complete blood lab; antigen lab; comprehensive allergy and chemical testing; detoxification saunas; nutritional counseling and education.

The Great Plains Laboratory, Inc.
11813 W 77th St.
Lenexa, KS 66214
(913) 341-8949
www.greatplainslaboratory.com
Vitamin and mineral deficiencies; organic acid test for yeast and bacteria overgrowth; opiate peptides for gluten and casein sensitivity; toxic exposures to heavy metals; deficiencies in the immune system; abnormal amino acids; comprehensive stool testing.

Great Smokies Diagnostic Laboratory
18A Regent Park Blvd.
Asheville, NC 28806
(704) 253-0621
www.gsdl.com
Amino acid analysis; essential and metabolic fatty acids; elemental analysis hair/urine test; comprehensive antibody assessment for food allergies.

[handwritten: GENOVA DIAGNOSTICS / www.GDX.NET 800-522-x762]

Immunosciences Laboratory Inc.
8730 Wilshire Blvd.
Beverly Hills, CA 90211
(310) 657-1077
www.immuno-sci-lab.com
Food allergy panels IgE and IgG; candida albanians antibiotic panel.

Metametrix Clinical Laboratory
4855 Peachtree Industrial Blvd.
Norcross, GA 30092
(800) 221-4640
www.metametrix.com
Fatty acids; amino acid profile; inhalant antibodies; toxic metals; IgE and IgG food antibodies.

Greenpeace Mercury Test Kit (hair analysis)
For $25.00
https://secureusa.greenpeace.org/mercury

Pain and Stress Center
5282 Medical Dr. #160
San Antonio, TX 78229-6043
(800) 669-CALM (2256)
www.painstresscenter.com
Nutritional counseling; amino acid testing; food allergy testing; ortho-
molecular programs; group lectures; educational programs
Product research and development

Q-Metrx Inc.   (QEEG)
1612 W. Olive Ave. Ste. 301
Burbank, CA 91506
(818) 563-5409
Info@q-metrx.com or www.q-metrx.com
Q-Metrx provides QEEG services nationally and internationally. The
Q-Metrx Processing center accepts digital EEGs sent through the
internet for expert analysis and interpretation.

MERCURY FREE DENTIST REFERRALS
International Academy of Oral Medicine and Toxicity
(407) 298-2450
www.iaomt.org

AMINO ACID SUPPLEMENTS AND OTHER NUTRIENTS
Apothecarey Pharmacy
11700 National Blvd.
Los Angeles, CA 90064
(310) 737-7277 or (866) 737-7277
www.apothecareypharmacy.net
Amino acids; Chinese herbs; compound pharmacy; Homeopathy.

Child Life Essentials
4051 Glencoe Ave., No. 11
Marine Del Rey, CA 90292
(800) 993-0332
www.childlife.net
Nutritional supplements for children and infants.

Longevity Medical Center, A Medical Corporation
2211 Corinth Ave. Ste. 204
Los Angeles, CA 90064
(310) 966-9194
www.drall.org
Amino acids supplements; nutritional supplements.

Metabolic Maintenance Products
P.O. Box 3600
Sisters, OR 97759
(800) 772-7873
www.metabolicmaintenance.com
Customized amino acid formula based on your profile from any reputable testing laboratory.

NeuroGenesis, Inc.
120 Park Ave.
League City, TX 77573
(800) 232-2583
www.neurogenesis.com
Neu•Becalm'd- Amino acid supplements.

NeuroResearch, Inc.
1150 88th Ave. W.
Duluth, MN 55808
(877) 626-2220
www.neuroreplete.com
Neurotransmitter testing; amino acid supplements.

Pain and Stress Center
5282 Medical Dr., No. 160
San Antonio, TX 78229-6043
(800) 669-CALM (2256)
www.painstresscenter.com
Amino acid supplements; nutritional supplements.

The Vitamin Shoppe
4700 Westside Ave.
North Bergen, NJ 07047
(800) 223-1216
www.VitaminShoppe.com
Amino acid supplements; nutritional supplements.

DETOX PRODUCTS
The American Botanical Pharmacy
P.O. Box 9699
Marina Del Rey, CA 90265
(800) 437-2362
www.herbdoc.com
Dr. Schulz Superfood; intestinal, liver/gallbladder and kidney/bladder detoxification herbal remedies.

BioRay, Inc.
NDF & NDF Plus
(888) 635-9582
www.Bioray2000.com
Organic dietary supplement for detoxifing heavy metals and chemicals.

CompliMed
1441 W. Smith Rd.
Ferndale, WA 98248
(888) 977-8008
www.complimed.com
Homeopathic detoxification products.

Health & Energy Alternatives
16915 SE 272nd St., Ste. 100, 226
Covington, WA 98042
(888) 235-1011
www.healternatives.com
Detoxification foot bath products.

RECOMMENDED HEALTH FOOD STORE PRODUCTS
ACIDOPHILUS
Bio-K+
www.biokplus.com
Promotes improved nutrient absorption. Reduces food sensitivity, by improving digestion and absorption. Enhances immune function.

ESSENTIAL FATTY ACIDS
Fish Oil
Carlson's
www.carlsonlabs.com

Health From the Sun
www.healthfromthesun.com

Nordic Naturals
www.nordicnaturals.com

Flaxseed Oil
Barlean's
www.barleans.com

Spectrum
www.spectrumorganics.com
Udo's Choice
www.udoerasmus.com

MINERALS
Trace Mineral Research
www.traceminerals.com

HOMEOPATHIC PRODUCTS
Hyland's
Calm Forte 4 Kids
www.hylands.com
A mild, non-addictive homeopathic remedy for promoting comfortable relaxation; contains chamomilla and hops.

Dr. Garber's Natural Solutions
Santa Monica, CA 90403
(310) 458-3223
www.drgarbers.com
Homeopathic Biotherapy Formulas for anxiety, allergies, depression, constipation, sleeplessness and other conditions.

RECOMMENDED WEBSITE
Free alternative health enewsletter
www.mercola.com

RECOMMENDED MAGAZINES
Alternative Medicine
www.alternativemedicine.com

Mothering
www.mothering.com

RECOMMENDED CLINICS
The HANDLE Institute
1300 Dexter Ave. N.
110 The Casey Family Building
Seattle, WA 98109
(206) 204-6000
www.handle.org
The HANDLE Institute provides an effective, non-drug alternative for identifying and treating most neurodevelopmental disorders across the lifespan including autism, ADD, ADHD, dyslexia and Tourette's syndrome.

Bibliography

DEBORAH MERLIN
Books

Prescriptions for Natural Healing
Balch, James F and Balch, Phyllis A (Avery Publishing Group, Inc.1990)
Talking Back To Ritalin
Breggin, Peter R. (Perseus Publishing 2001)
The Yeast Connection—A Medical Breakthrough
Crook, William G. (Vintage Books 1983)
A Shot In The Dark
Coulter, Harris L. (Avery 1991)
The Body Ecology Diet
Gates, Donna (B.E.D. Publications 1996)
Alternative Health, the Definitive Guide,
Goldberg, Burton Group (Future Medicine Publishing Inc. 1994)
Crimes Against Nature
Kennedy, Robert F., Jr. (Harper Collins Publishers 2004)
Complete Candida Yeast Guidebook
Martin, Jeanne Marie (Prima Publishing 1996)
Born too Soon
Mehren, Elizabeth (Doubleday 1991)
Total wellness
Pizzorno, Joseph (Prima Publishing 1996)
Is This Your Child? Discovering and Treating Unrecognized Allergies
Rapp, Doris (William Morrow and Company, Inc. 1991)
Control Hyperactivity
Sahley, Billie Jay (Pain and Stress Publications 1994)
Heal with Amino Acids and Nutrients
Sahley, Billie Jay (Pain & Stress Publications 2001)
The Yeast Syndrome
Trowbridge, John Parks (Bantam Books 1986)
Natural Treatments for ADD and Hyperactivity
Weintraub, Syke (Woodland Publishing 1997)

Dental Mercury Detox
   Ziff, Sam (Bio Probe, Inc. 1988)

Additonal Sources
- www.Addhelpsite.com/sideeffects.htm, ADD help site
- www.add-adhd-kids.com/depakote.html
- *Nine Steps to Detox from Mercury Fillings* (Alternative Healing Magazine, Issue 29, May, 1999)
- Johnson, Jack, www.q-Metrx.com
- *Safety Lead Levels Lower IQ in Children*, Study Finds (Los Angeles Times, April 17, 2003)
- *Early Help Cuts Premature Babies, Risk*, Study Finds (Los Angeles Times, June, 1990)
- *Your Health and Dairy Products,* (Quality Longevity, Lovendale, Mark, 1993)
- *Vaccine Fillers and Ingredients* (www.Mercola.com 1997-2003)
- *Vaccines and Autism* (Mothering magazine, November, 2002)
- *Are Everyday Chemicals Harming Our Children* (Moyer, Bill, KCET, NOW, 2002)
- *Children's Chemical and Pesticide Exposure via Food Products* (The National Academies Advisors to the Nation of Science, Engineering, and Medicine U.S. Government Facts Products, July, 2005)
- *Depakote Side Effects* (Public Citizens eLetter www.citizens.org. & www.adhd-kids.com October, 2000)
- *Artificial Food Coloring and Food Allergies Information for Parents* (www.Safechild.net)
- *Biological Treatments for Autism and PDD* (Shaw, William, Ph.D., The Great Plains Laboratory, Inc. 2002)
- *Self Healing Newsletter* (Weil Andrew, M.D., September, 2002)

LARRY COOK
Basic Macrobiotics
   Aihara, Herman (Japan Publications, Inc. 1991)
Cleanse & Purify Thyself
   Anderson, Richard (Anderson, 1994)
Against the Grain
   Bailey, Britt and Lappe, Marc (The Tides Center / CETOS 1998)

Prescription for Nutritional Healing
    Balch, James and Phyllis (Avery Publishing Group 1997)
Alkalize or Die
    Baroody, Theodore (Holographic Health Press 1991)
The Eco-Foods Guide
    Barstow, Cynthia (New Society Publishers 2002)
Excitotoxins—The Taste that Kills
    Blaylock, Russell (Health Press 1997)
Apple Cider Vinegar, Miracle Health System
    Bragg, Patricia and Paul (Health Science)
Herbal Prescriptions for Better Health
    Brown, Donald (Prima Publishing 1996)
Silent Spring
    Carson, Rachel (Houghton Mifflin Company 1994)
Our Stolen Future
    Colborn, Theo & Dumanoski, Dianne & Myers, John (PLUME 1997)
Sugar Blues
    Dufty, William (Warner Books 1975)
Eating With Conscience
    Fox, Michael (NewSage Press 1997)
Get the Sugar Out
    Gittleman, Ann Louise (Three Rivers Press 1996)
Overcoming Parasites
    Gittleman, Ann Louise (Avery Publishing Group 1999)
An Introduction to Macrobiotics
    Heidenry, Carolyn (Avery Publishing Group 1992)
Vitamin B-3 & Schizophrenia
    Hoffer, Abram (Quary Press, Inc. 1998)
Immunization: The Reality Behind the Myth
    James, Walene (Bergin & Garvey 1995)
Natural Healing through Macrobiotics
    Kushi, Michio (Japan Publications, Inc. 1978)
The Medical Mafia
    Lanctot, Guylaine (Here's the Key, Inc. 1995)
Chemical Deception
    Lappe, Marc (Sierra Club Books 1991)

Mad Cowboy
Lyman, Howard (Touchstone 1998)
Wheat Grass – Nature's Finest Medicine
Meyerowitz, Steve (Sproutman Publications 1999)
Encyclopedia of Nutritional Supplements
Murray, Michael (Prima Publishing 1996)
Practical Guide to Natural Medicines
Peirce, Andrea (The Stonesong Press, Inc. 1999)
Healing with Whole Foods
Pitchford, Paul (North Atlantic Books 1993)
Diet for a New America
Robbins, John (Stillpoint Publishing 1987)
The Food Revolution
Robbins, John (Conari Press 2001)
Reclaiming Our Health
Robbins, John (HJ Krammer, Inc. 1996)
In Bad Taste
Schwartz, George (Health Press 1999)
Seeds of Deception
Smith, Jeffrey (YES! Books, 2003)
Why Can't I Eat That!
Taylor, John F. and Latta, Sharon R. (ADD-Plus 1996)
The Encyclopedia of Natural Remedies
Tebbey, Louise (Woodland Publishing, Inc. 1995)
Genetically Engineered Foods
Ticciati, Laura and Robin (Keats Publishing, Inc. 1998)
Elements of Danger
Walker, Morton (Hamptom Roads Publishing Company, Inc. 2000)
The Natural Way to Vibrant Health
Walker, Norman (Norwalk Press 1972)
Food Irradiation
Webb, Tony/ Lang, Tim/ Tucker, Kathleen (Thorsons Publishers, Inc. 1987)
Fateful Harvest
Wilson, Duff (HarperCollins 2001)
Genetically Engineered Food: Changing the Nature of Nature
Wilson, Kimberly (Park Street Press 1999)

Notes

3. The Problems with Conventional Medicine

[1] See Chapter 6 for more information.

[2] See Chapter 7 for more information.

[3] Walene James, *Immunization: The Reality Behind the Myth* (Westport, CT: Greenwood Press, 1995), 43.

[4] Ibid., 235.

[5] Ibid., 108.

[6] If you choose to vaccinate, the best time to do so is when your child is healthy. If the child is sick or has a weakened immune system, consider arranging a different time for the vaccination. Furthermore, immediately prior to and after vaccination, ample amounts of Vitamin C is highly recommended.

4. Why Ritalin Isn't the Answer

[1] Mary Eberstadt, "Why Ritalin Rules," *Policy Review* No. 94 April/May 1999. www.policyreview.org/apr99/eberstadt.html.

[2] "Ritalin: Violence against boys: Drug is being used to sedate active, young boys," *Massachusetts News* (Marlborough, MA) 1 November 1999.

[1] U.S. Drug Enforcement Administration, "News Release: Methylphenidate," 20 October 1995. www.dea.gov/pubs/pressrel/pr951020.htm.

[2] Ibid.

[3] William J. Bailly, Indiana Prevention Resource Center (Indiana University), "Factline on Non-Medical Use of Ritalin," *Factline* No. 9 November 1995. www.onelife.com/edu/indiana.html.

[4] *Physician's Desk Reference* (Montvale, NJ: Medical Economics Co., 1995).

[5] National Institutes of Health, "Diagnosis and Treatment of Attention Deficit Hyperactivity Disorder: Consensus Development Conference Statement," 16–18 November 1998. http://consensus.nih.gov/1998/1998AttentionDeficitHyperactivityDisorder110html.htm.

[6] "A Dose of Reality," *Adbusters* July/August 2001, 16.

[7] Fact sheet from Eli Lilly, the drug's manufacturer. Available online at www.strattera.com/1_2_taking_strattera/1_2_4_safety.jsp.

[8] Consider also the perspective on behavioral problems, including attention disorders, offered by The HANDLE Institute, discussed at www.handle.org and described in Chapter 5.

[9] "Kids Are Suffering Legal Drug Abuse," *The Boston Globe* 26 September 1999.

[10] "A Dose of Reality," 16

[11] "The Business of ADHD," *Frontline* (PBS) April 2001.

[12] Ibid.

5. Attentional Priority Disorder—Not Attention Deficit Disorder

[1] The HANDLE Institute treats a range of neurological issues, including, but not limited to, attention disorders, autism, learning disabilities, Tourette's syndrome, and brain injury. It addresses these challenges with an individualized neurodevelopmental profile, recommendations of ways to improve nutrition, and a personalized program of gentle "organized movement" activities. To contact HANDLE, visit www.handle.org or call the institute's Seattle headquarters at (206) 204-6000.

[2] Judith Bluestone speaking on "The HANDLE Approach," taken from a recording of an informational community seminar in 1997.

[3] All information, whether taken in by hearing, sight, touch or another sense, travels through and among the nervous system circuitry via neurons. The sheath around a neuron's axon consists of myelin, which insulates the axon. The thicker the myelin, the faster the messages travel across the neuron. Myelin is created in the presence of essential fatty acids. Therefore, as HANDLE notes, a diet that includes these fatty acids, specifically omega-3 fatty acids, is important for efficient nervous-system functioning. Omega-3 fatty acids can be obtained from cold-processed flaxseed oil as well as fish oil derived from salmon, mackerel, cod and other cold-water fish. (Read Chapter 7 for additional information about essential fatty acids.)

[4] Both problems are addressed by HANDLE primarily through gentle "organized movement" activities, described in further detail at the end of this chapter and at the institute's Web site.

6. Possible Causes of Neurological Disorders

[1] Information in this section is based on three sources (which contain additional extensive citations and references):

1. Herman Aihara, *Basic Macrobiotics* (New York: Japan Publications, Inc., 1985).

2. John Robbins, *Diet For a New America: How Your Food Choices Affect Your Health, Happiness and the Future of Life on Earth* (Tiburon, CA: H J Kramer, 1998).

3. People for the Ethical Treatment of Animals, "Vegan Children: Healthy and Happy." www.peta.org/mc/factsheet_display.asp?ID=100.

² Paul Pitchford, *Healing with Whole Foods: Asian Traditions and Modern Nutrition* (Berkeley: North Atlantic Books, 2002), 32.

² Award-winning investigative reporter Christopher Bryson, in his book, *The Fluoride Deception* (Seven Stories Press, 2004), describes in detail the part fluoride played during the development of the atomic bomb, subsequent cover-ups, and the foisting of this substance on the American public.

³ Fluoride Action Network, "Dental Fluorosis." 25 August 2005. www.fluoridealert.org/dental-fluorosis.htm.

⁴ Ibid., "Facts About Fluoridation." March 2002. www.fluoridealert.org/fluoride-facts.htm.

⁵ Ibid., "Health Effects: Fluoride & Tooth Decay (Caries)." www.fluoridealert.org/health/teeth/caries/index.html.

⁶ Neurotoxicity is defined as adverse effects on the structure or function of the central and/or peripheral nervous system caused by exposure to a toxic chemical. Symptoms of neurotoxicity include muscle weakness, loss of sensation and motor control, tremors, cognitive alterations, and autonomic nervous system dysfunction. For more information, see www.trufax.org/general/chemical.html.

⁷ Morton Walker and Julian Whitaker, *Elements of Danger: Protect Yourself Against the Hazards of Modern Dentistry* (Charlottesville, VA: Hampton Roads Publishing Company, 1999), 135.

⁸ Sallie Bernard, A. Enayati, L. Redwood, H. Roger, and T. Binstock, ARC Research, "Autism: A Novel Form of Mercury Poisoning." www.mercola.com/2000/oct/1/autism_mercury.htm. For more information, contact ARC Research, 14 Commerce Dr., Cranford, NJ 07901; (908) 276-6300 (phone) and (908) 276-1301 (fax).

⁹ Matthew Shaffer, "Waste Lands: The Threat of Toxic Fertilizer." 3 May 2001. http://pirg.org/toxics/reports/wastelands/index.html.

[10] Animal products accumulate these toxins in their fat, and the accumulated amounts are passed on to those who eat meat.

[11] Robbins, 321.

[12] Environmental Working Group (www.ewg.org). This group does an excellent job of citing their sources of information, often from government agencies.

[13] Marc Lappe, *Chemical Deception: The Toxic Threat to Health and the Environment* (San Francisco: Sierra Club Books, 1991), 86-87.

[14] Richard Alexander, "Birth Defects Caused by Herbicides, Insecticides, and Industrial Chemicals that Disrupt the Endocrine System," *The Consumer Law Page*. http://consumerlawpage.com/article/endocrine.shtml.

[15] Endocrine toxicity is defined as any adverse structural and/or functional changes to the endocrine system (the system that controls hormones in the body) that may result from exposure to chemicals. Endocrine toxicity can harm human and animal reproduction and development. For more information, see www.trufax.org/general/chemical.html.

[16] T. Colborn, F. Vom Saal, and P. Short, eds., "Environmental Endocrine-Disrupting Chemicals: Neural, Endocrine, and Behavioral Effects," *Princeton Scientific Publishing* (1998): 1–9. The report is available at www.worldwildlife.org/toxics/pubs/con_5.htm.

[17] Christopher S. Kilham, *The Bread & Circus Whole Food Bible: How to Select and Prepare Safe, Healthful Foods Without Pesticides or Chemical Additives* (Upper Saddle River, NJ: Addison Wesley Longman Publishing, 1991), 4.

[18] Ben F. Feingold, *Why Your Child Is Hyperactive* (New York: Random House, 1996).

[19] Renee Sharp and Sonya Lunder, Environmental Working Group, "High Levels of Toxic Fire Retardants Contaminate American Homes." www.ewg.org/reports/inthedust/summary.php.

7. Nontoxic Solutions

[1] Paul Pitchford, *Healing with Whole Foods: Asian Traditions and Modern Nutrition* (Berkeley: North Atlantic Books, 2002), 188–189.

[2] Richard Anderson, *Cleanse & Purify Thyself* (Medford, OR: Christobe Publishing, 2000), 10.

[3] Note: Naturopaths are trained in homeopathy, but not all homeopathic practitioners are naturopaths.

About the Authors

Deborah Merlin

For fifteen years Deborah Merlin made it her mission to be an advocate for her children's special needs. A new mother of very premature twins with challenging health problems, she found that doctors and other professionals offered only drugs as the solution. To find alternative ways to heal her children she attended alternative medicine and nutritional seminars, performed extensive research on ADHD and other health-related issues, and kept impeccable records.

In 1993, she was the co-chair of the Westside Cities Council to help promote Public Law 99457, part H, which implemented early intervention services from birth through three years of age for children at risk. She co-ran a parent support group at the Westside Regional Center in Culver City, California, that focused on children with special needs and those at risk.

In 1990 and 1991, she was the coordinator for Outreach to Pediatricians (under Public Law 99457, part H) and coordinated presentations at hospitals to educate pediatricians on early intervention services and resources for children at risk from infancy to three years of age. She was a guest speaker on radio programs to promote early intervention.

She was employed by Equifax Services as an insurance investigator from 1977 to 1991, which helped develop her research and analytical skills.

She is also an artist.

Larry Cook

Larry has successfully launched, published, and sold two magazines devoted to natural living. He converted his publishing experience and research into his recently published book, *The Beginner's Guide to Natural Living* (www.TheNaturalGuide.com). *Victory Over ADHD* reflects his extensive study of holistic ADHD treatments. Larry, a location sound mixer in Hollywood for TV-related projects, is currently developing his next release: a natural living DVD video. He lives in Los Angeles.

Order Information

To order a copy of *Victory Over ADHD*, please:

1. Send check or money order for $20 to:

   Deborah Merlin
   10008 National Blvd., Ste. 439
   Los Angeles, CA 90034

   Include your name, address and phone number.

OR

2. Go to www.VictoryOverADHD.com and place your order on our web site.

Thank you!